WELLNESS HABITS MAZE

TO:

FROM:

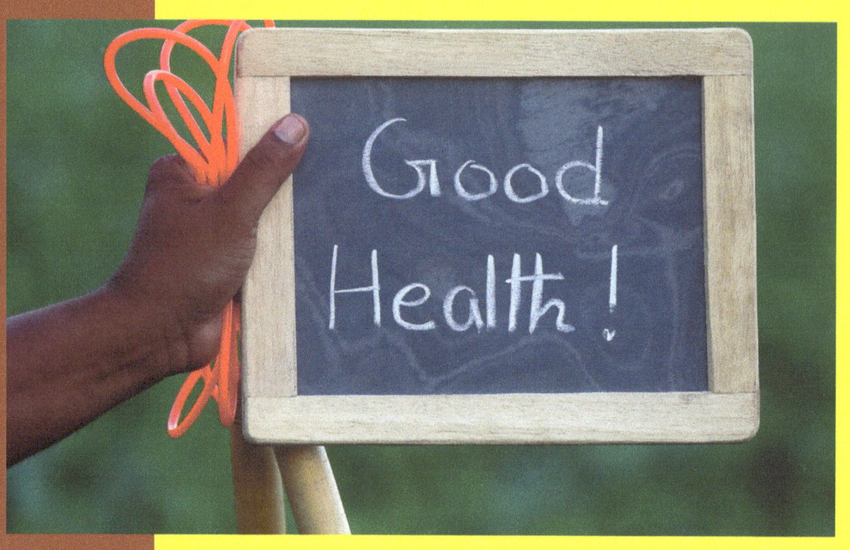

JOY VIZANTE

Our Wellness Maze is a reminder to stay well – mind, body and soul.

ALL MAZES LEAD TO THE CENTER OR EXIT TO THE SIDE!

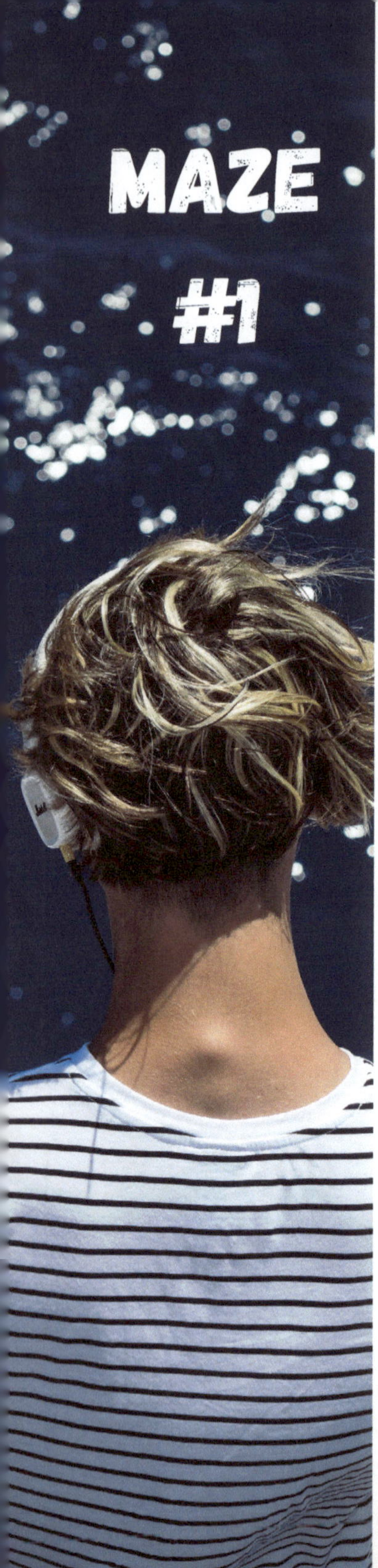

CAN YOU WALK AND TALK?

Have a meeting coming up soon or an important conversation? Put on a pair of headphones and stroll fo at least 30-minutes if possible. This will revive your body and mind.

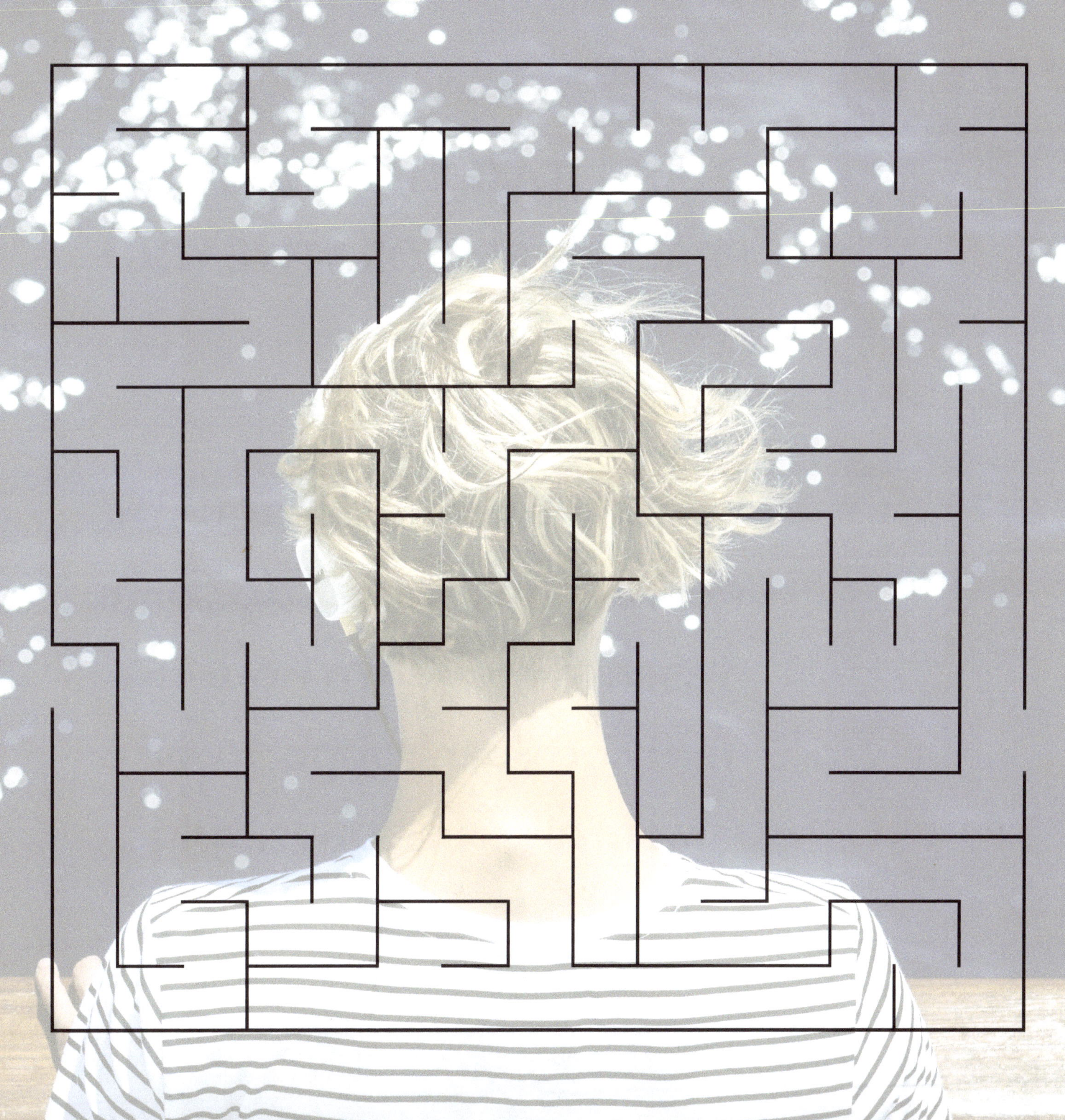

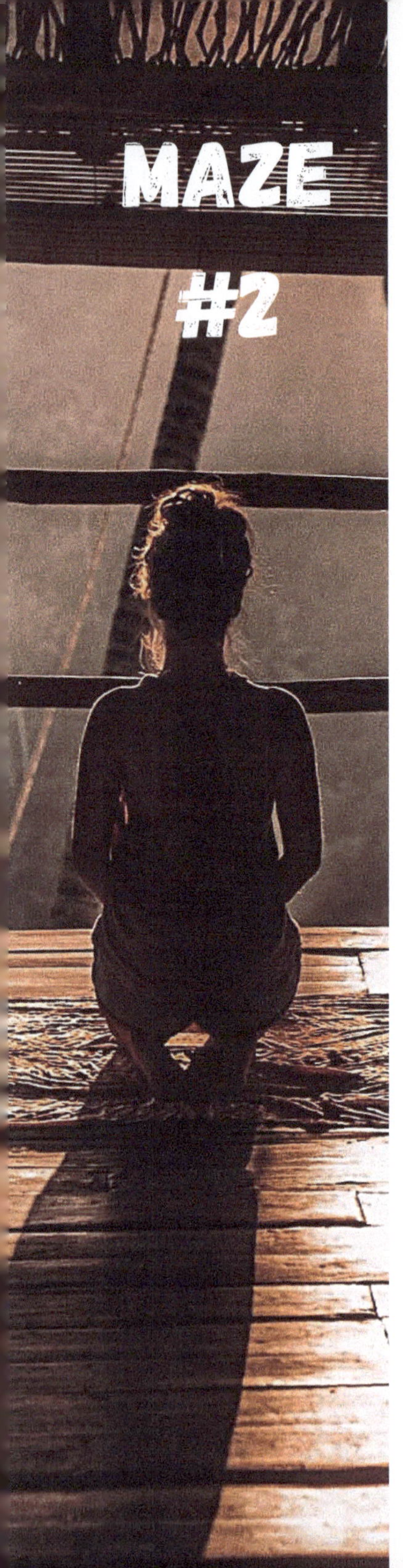

TAKE TİME TO PRACTİCE RESTORATİVE YOGA

If you're not familiar with Restorative yoga, do some research to learn how the methods can support you - mentally and physically.

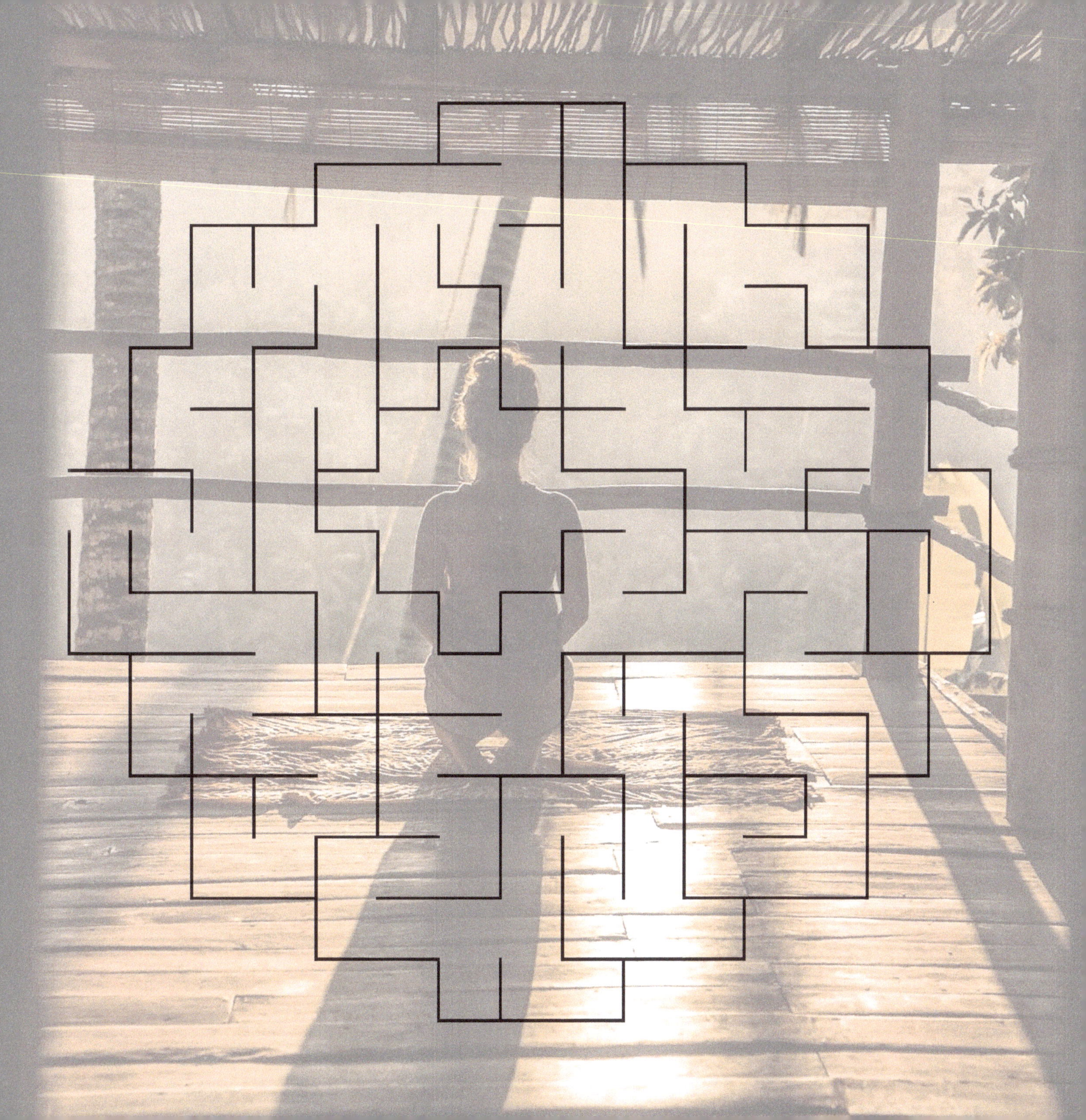

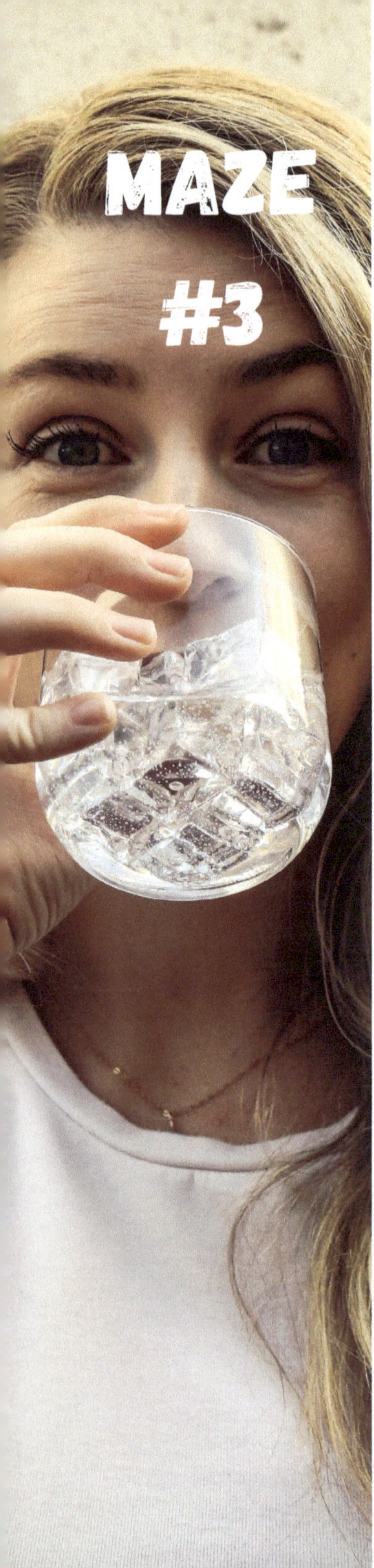

DRİNK MORE WATER

Keep a large bottle of water on your desk and make a point to fill it to help you maintain hydration and support your well-being.

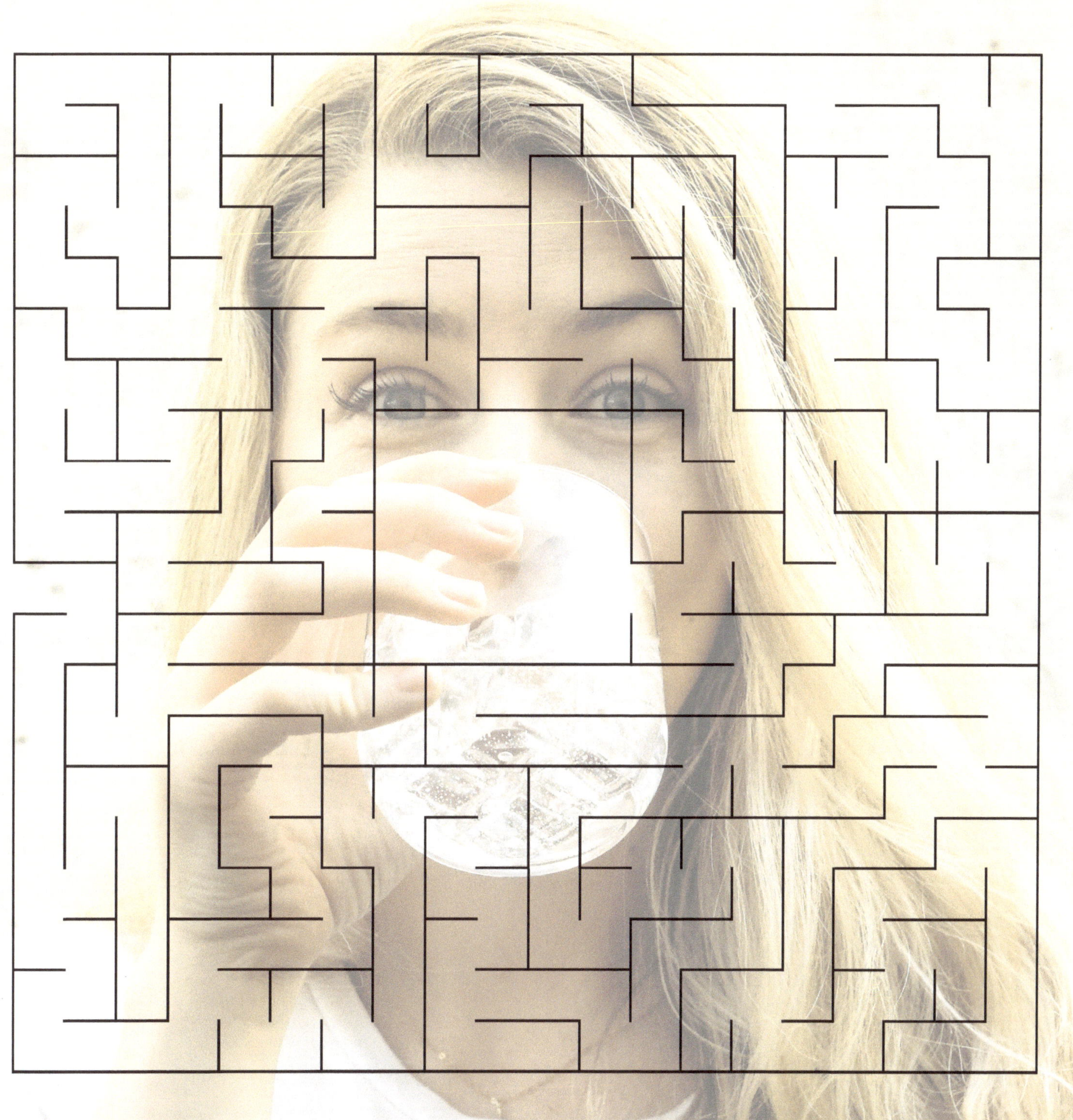

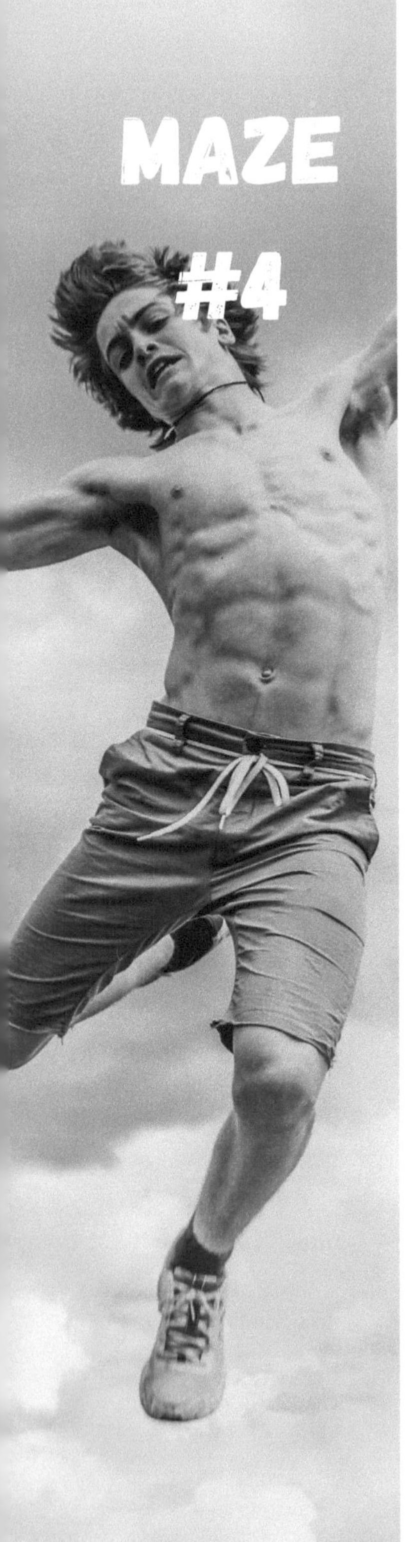

LİSTEN TO YOUR BODY'S SİGNALS

Try to look out for signals from your body. This can help you relax and rest when you need to. We often push overselves but there are times your body will enjoy a break of relaxation.

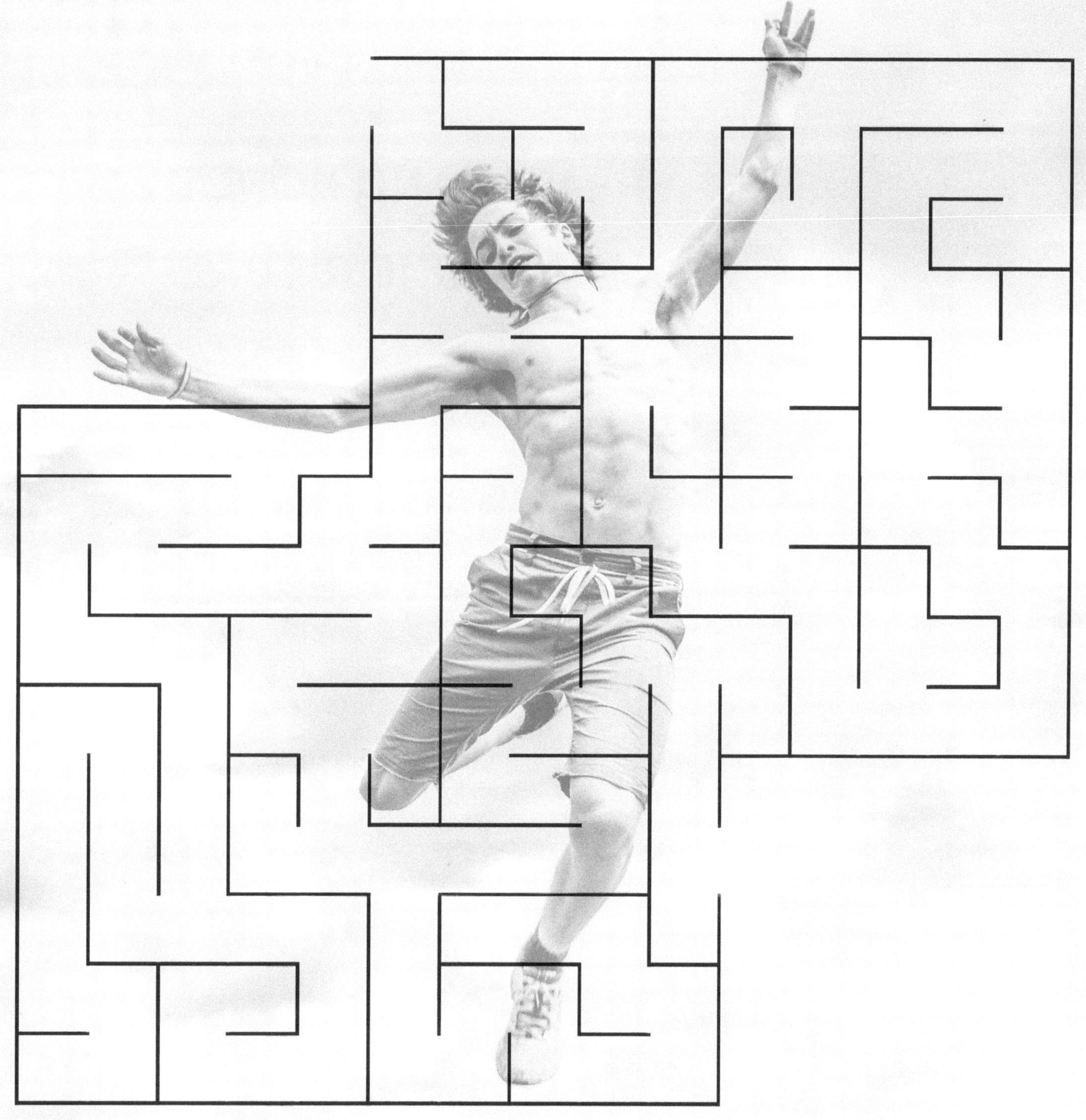

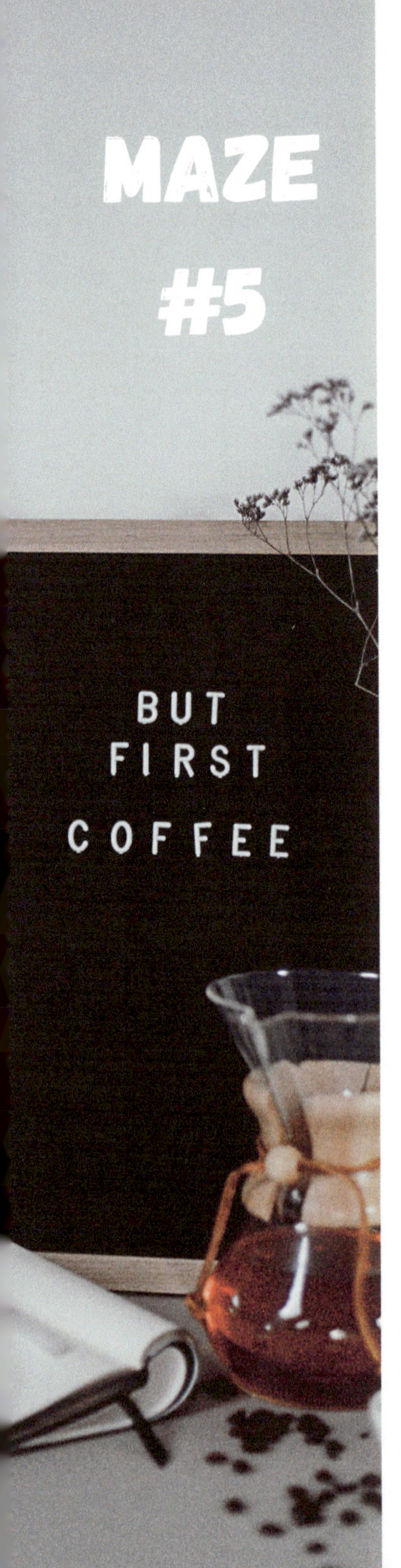

CREATE (AND HONOR) A MORNING RITUAL

A great way to set yourself up for success is by establishing a morning routine. This is not just for work, you can start this even before your workday has started.

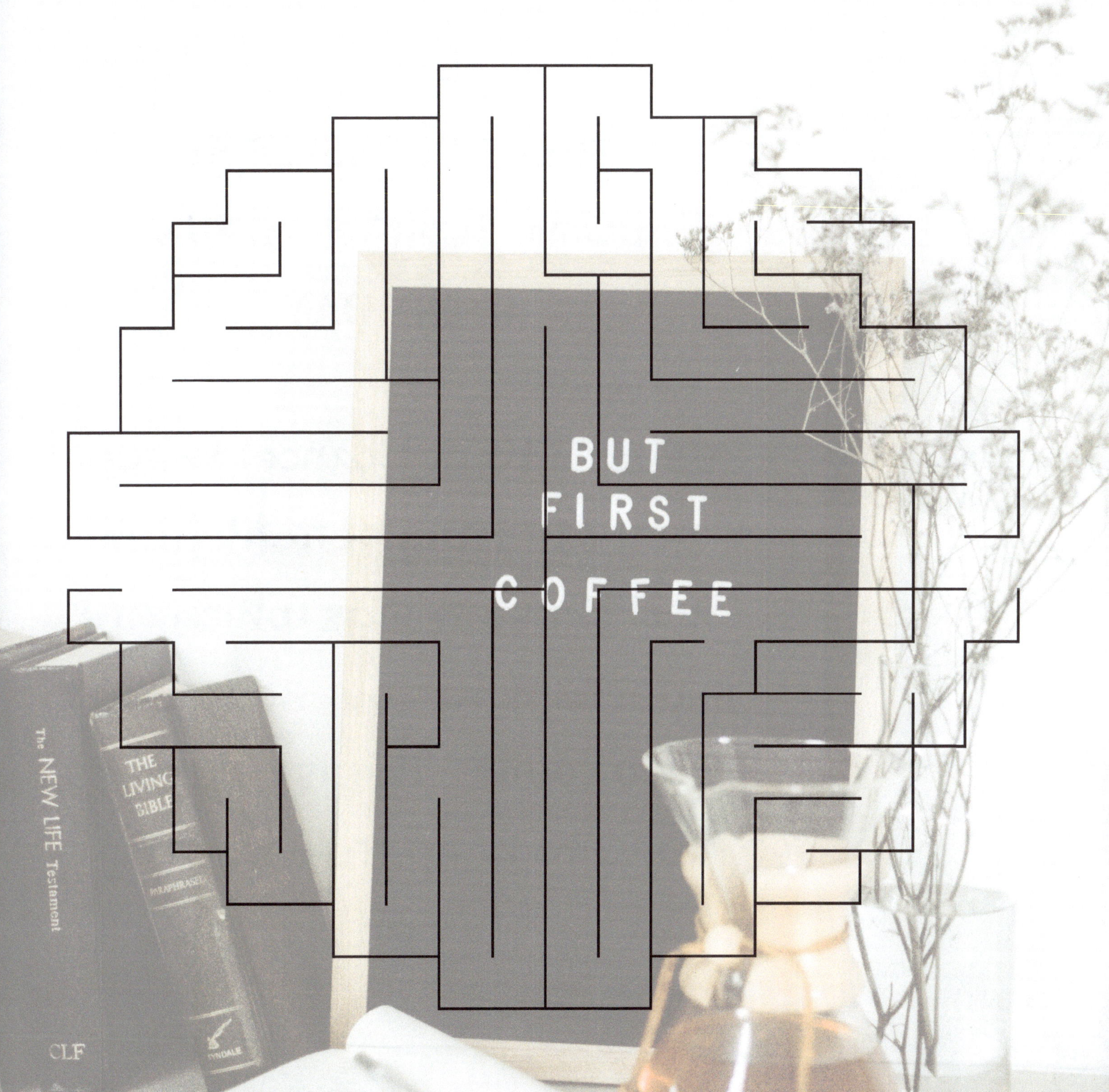

BUT
FIRST
COFFEE
The NEW LIFE Testament
THE LIVING BIBLE
PARAPHRASED
CLF
TYNDALE

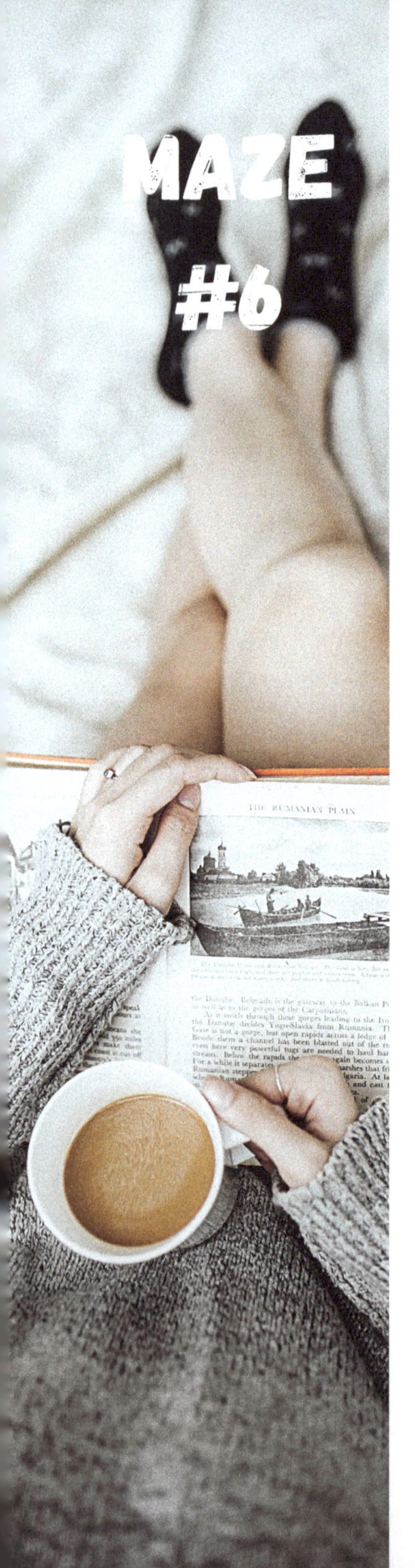

TREAT YOURSELF BY DOİNG SOMETHİNG FUN EVERY DAY

Be sure to not cancel things you can truly benefit from and those things which are important to you. Remember you count. This is a great way to keep from burning out!

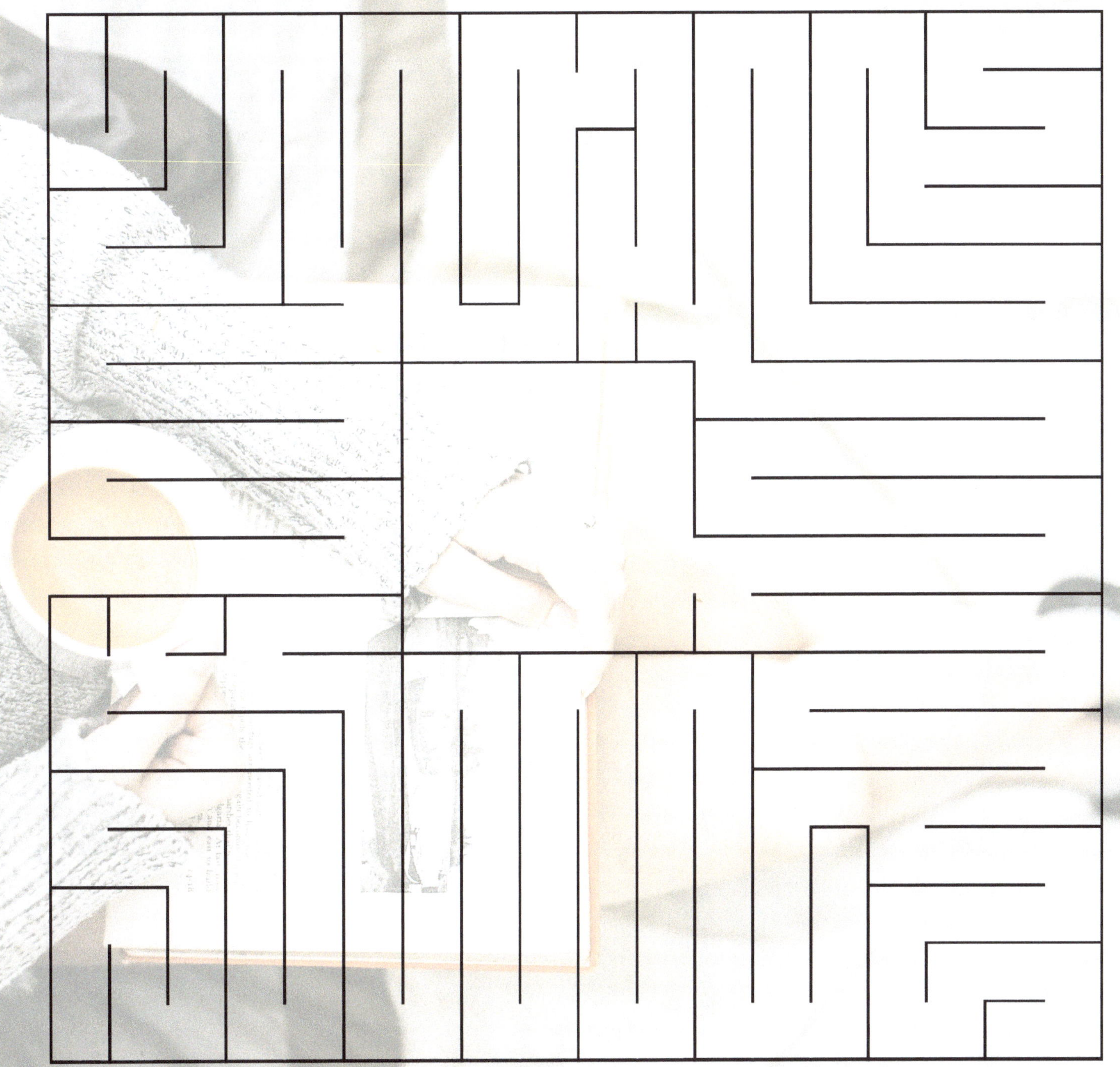

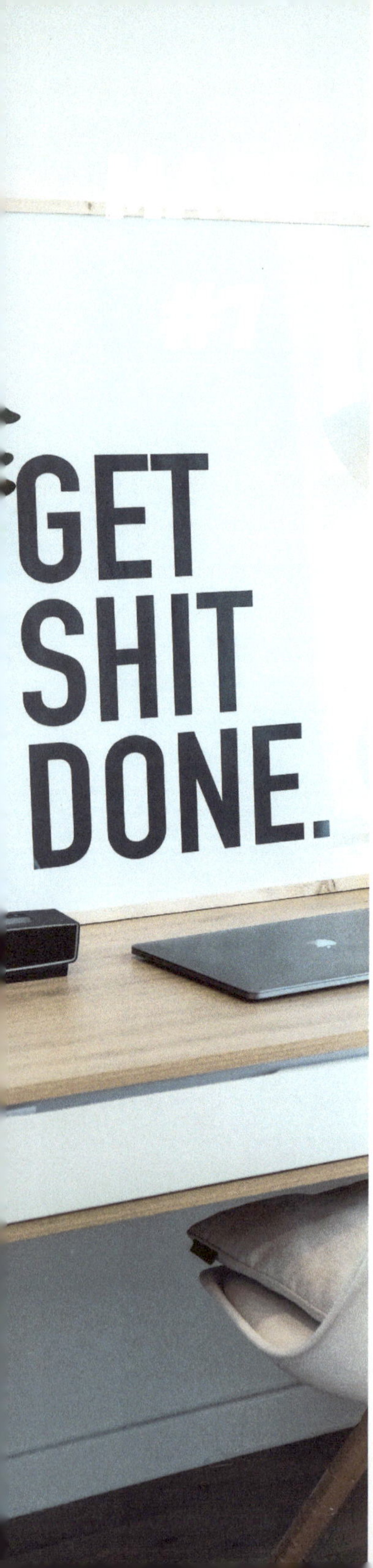

SET BOUNDARIES WITH WORK —AND COMMIT TO THEM

Each day we're all met with different demands throughout the day, however, commit to a firm boundary when necessary. Sometimes we need space which actually may help with doing the job well.

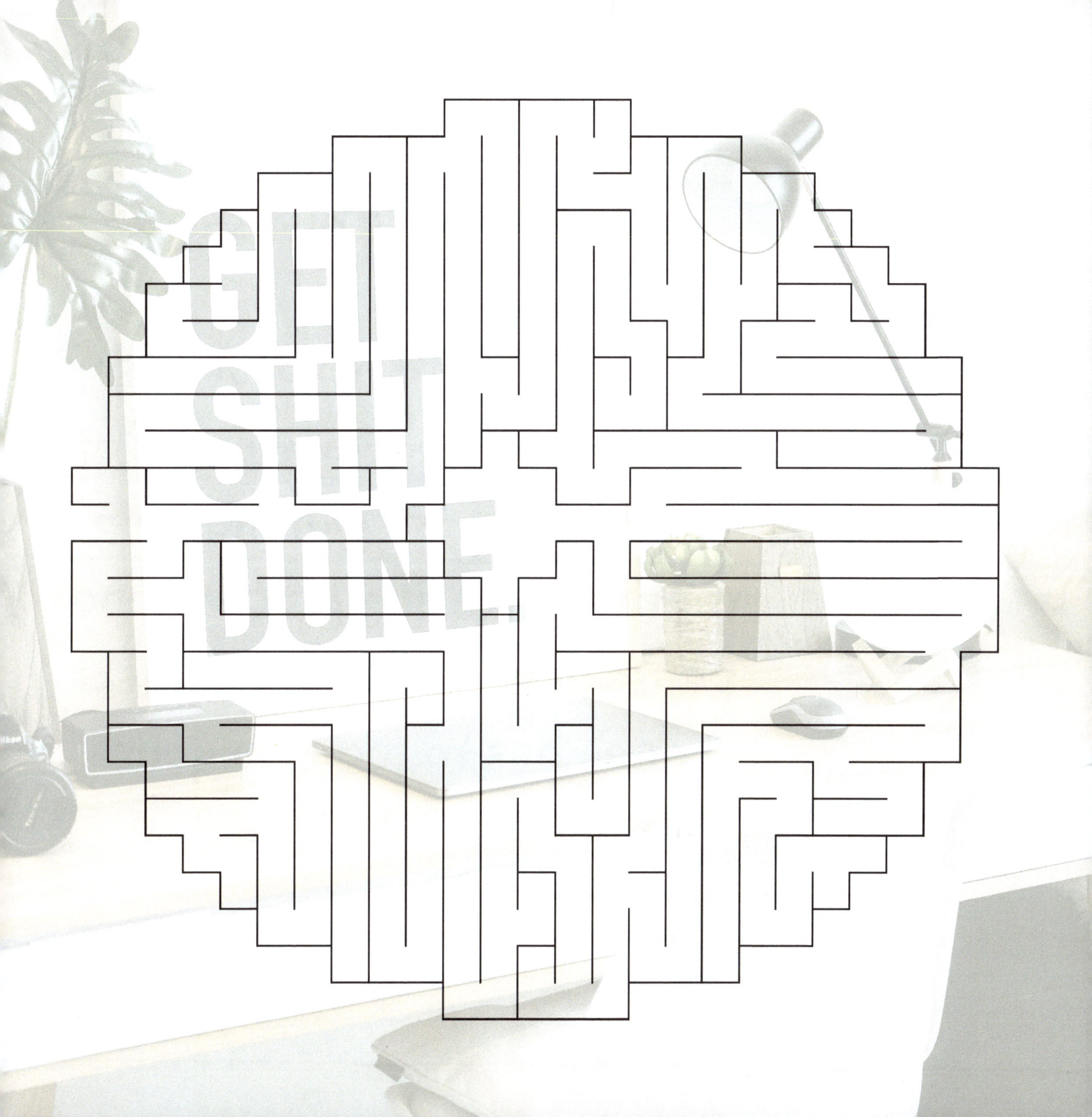

GET
SHIT
DONE.

GİVE MEDİTATİON A SHOT

You can practice mindfulness ys simply adding five minutes of meditation to your morning routine or taking a 60-second pause in between work tasks or emails to focus on your breath and to recenter yourself.

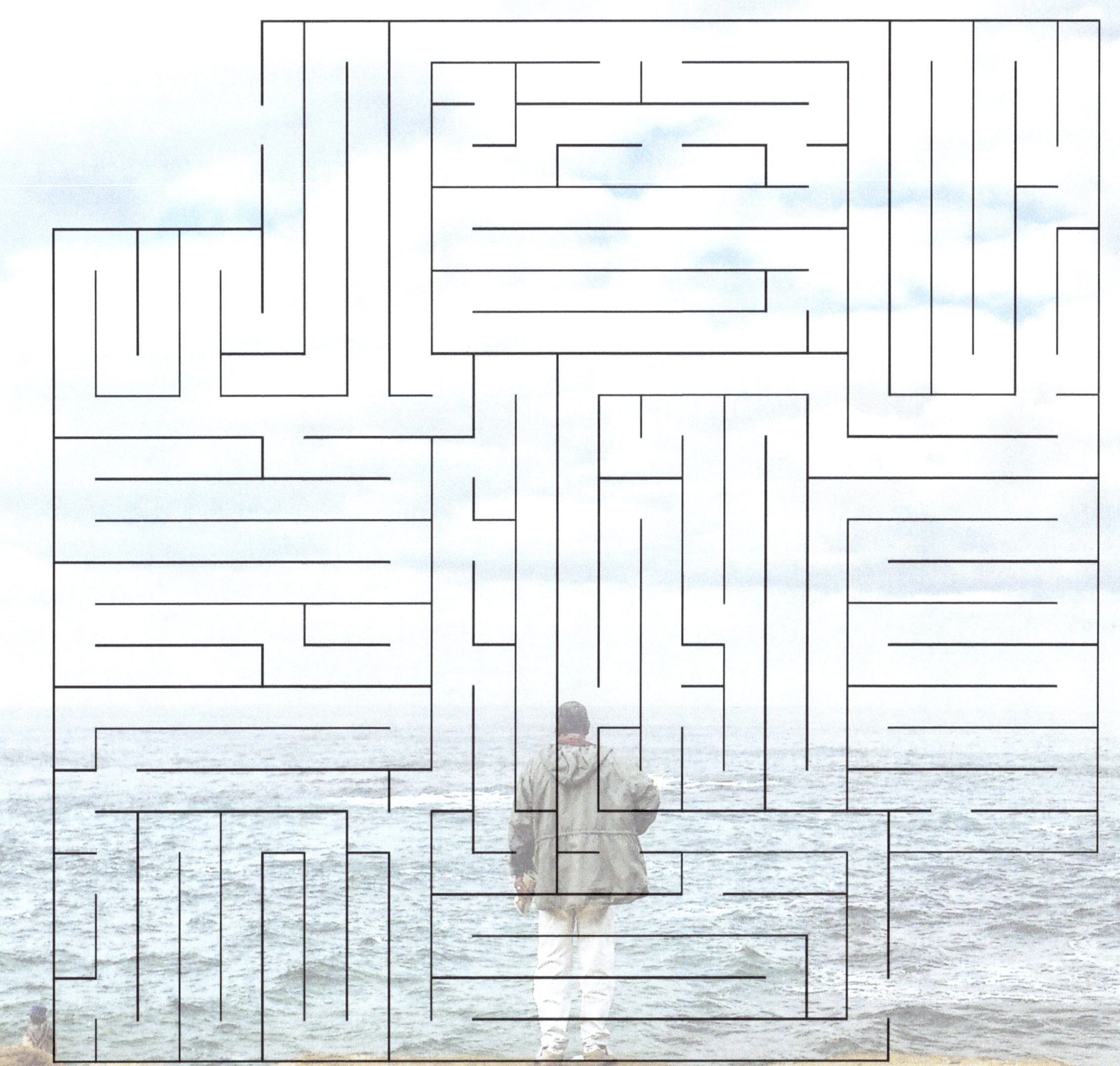

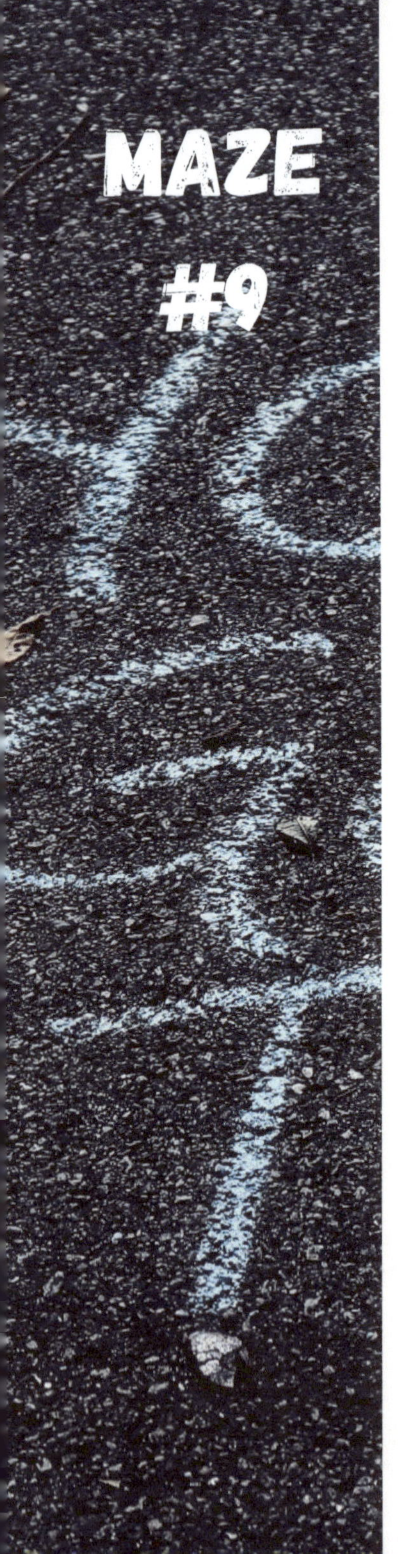

LEAD WITH A POWER MANTRA

An examples is stating something like: 'I am highly successful in whatever I choose to do,' or 'There is nothing too big for me to handle with ease.' These type of affirmations can set the tone for the entire day.

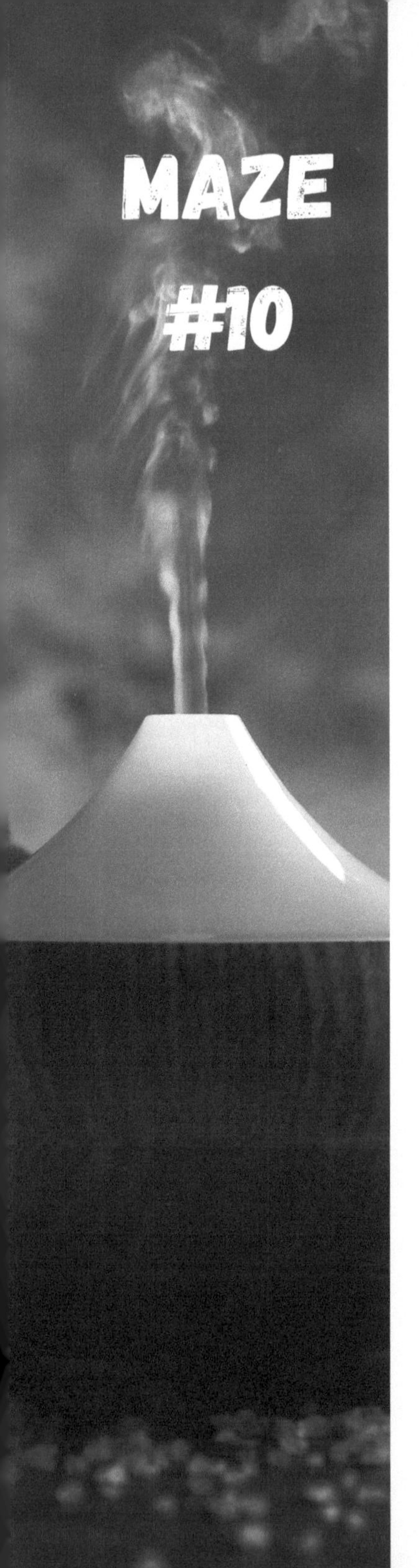

INDULGE THE SENSES
WITH AROMATHERAPY

Incorporating essential oils into your office space, or a nighttime or morning routine can add a moment of wellness and help you destress from a busy or hectic day.

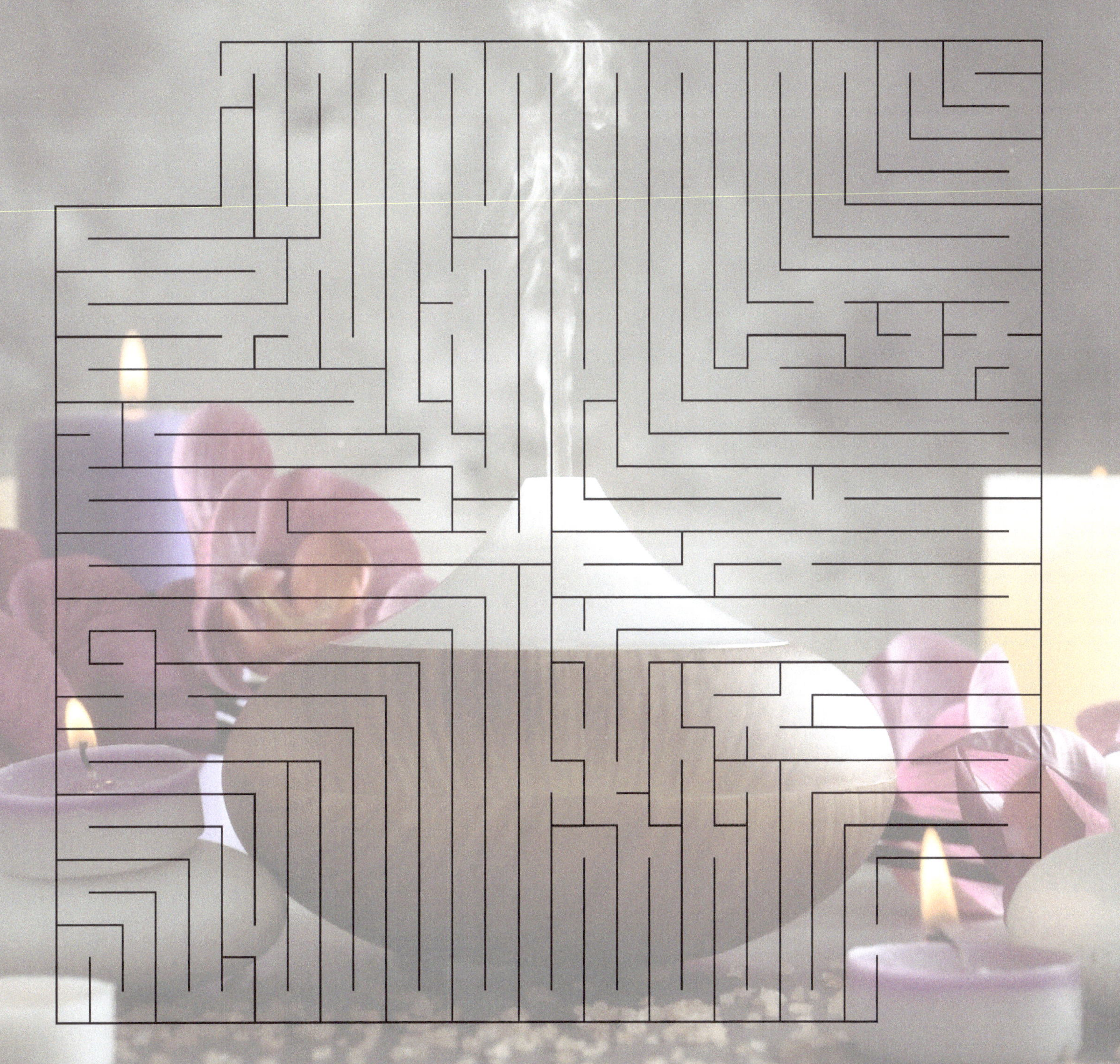

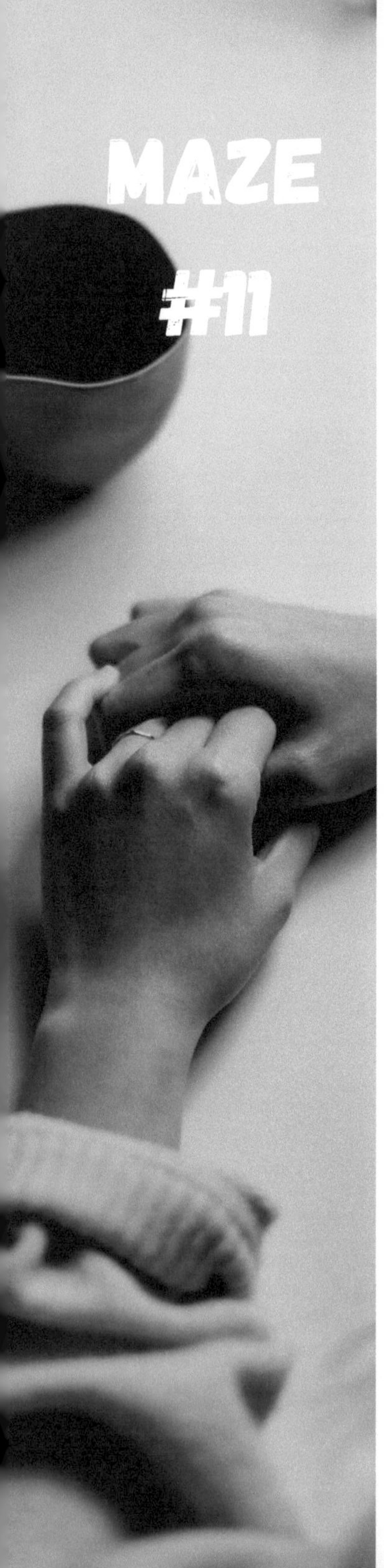

MAKE A HABIT OF MEANINGFUL CONVERSATIONS

Look for opportunites to communicate with those who matter to you! Take breaks to check in with yourself as well as others who bring you peace.

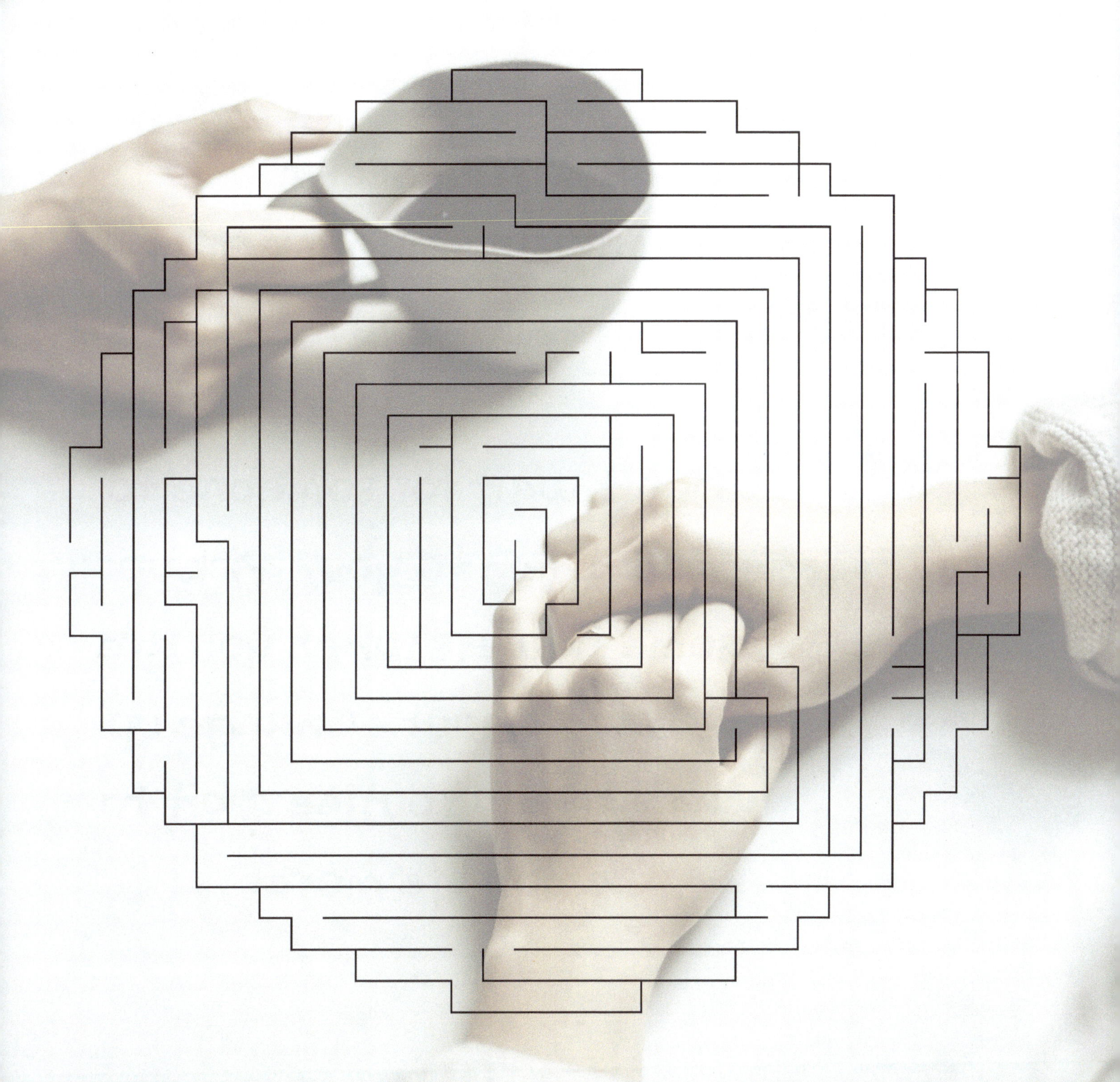

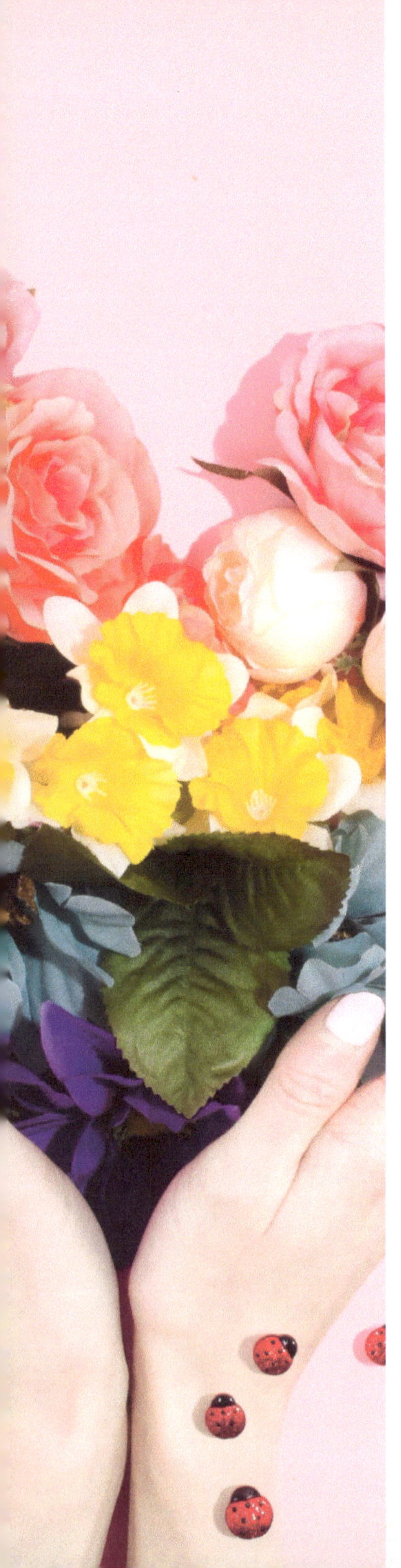

BUY YOURSELF A
BEAUTIFUL BOUQUET OF
FLOWERS

Don't wait for someone to give them to you. Pick up some flowers when you are out and about. Change up habits and routine a bit to enjoy life more.

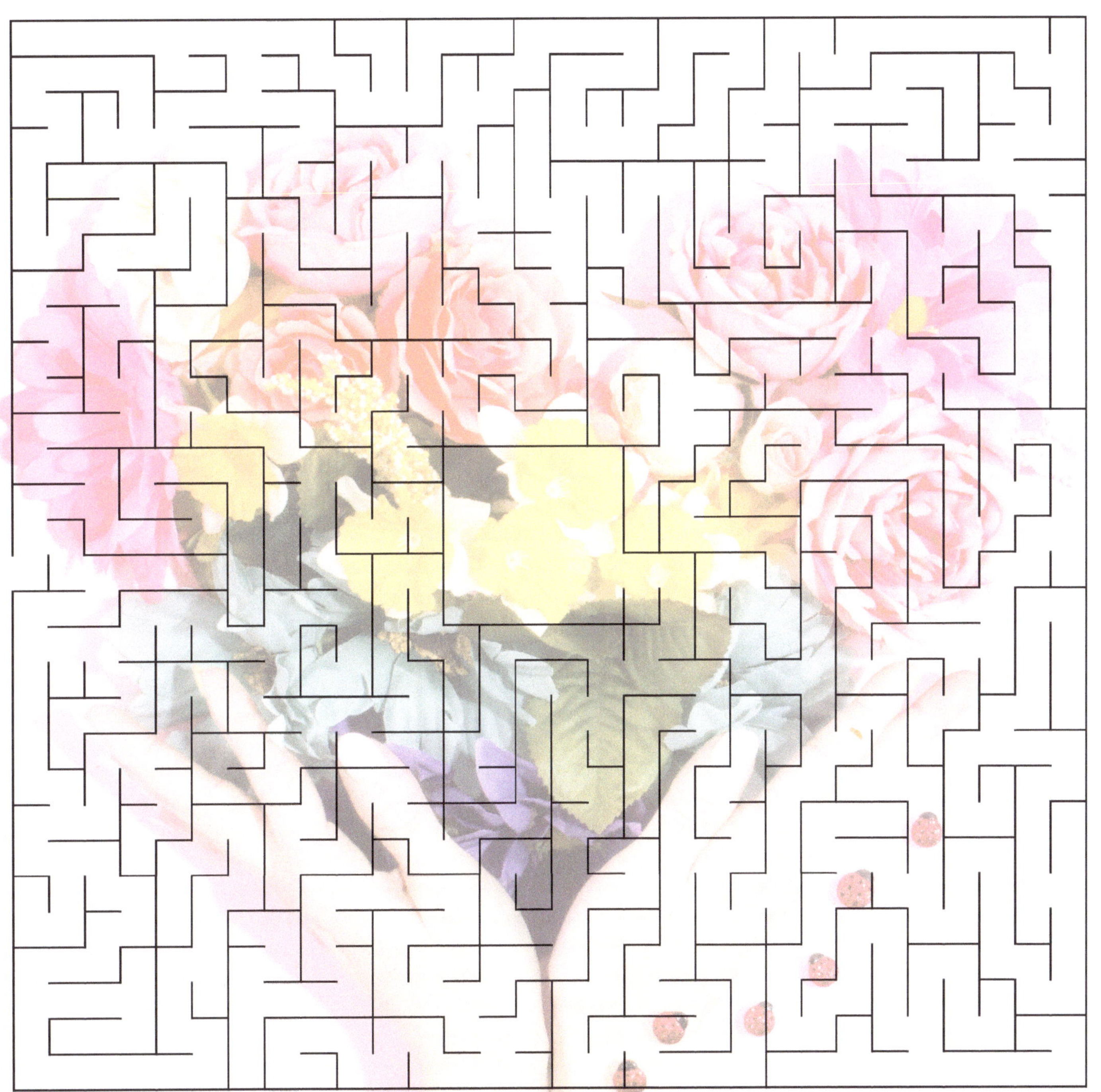

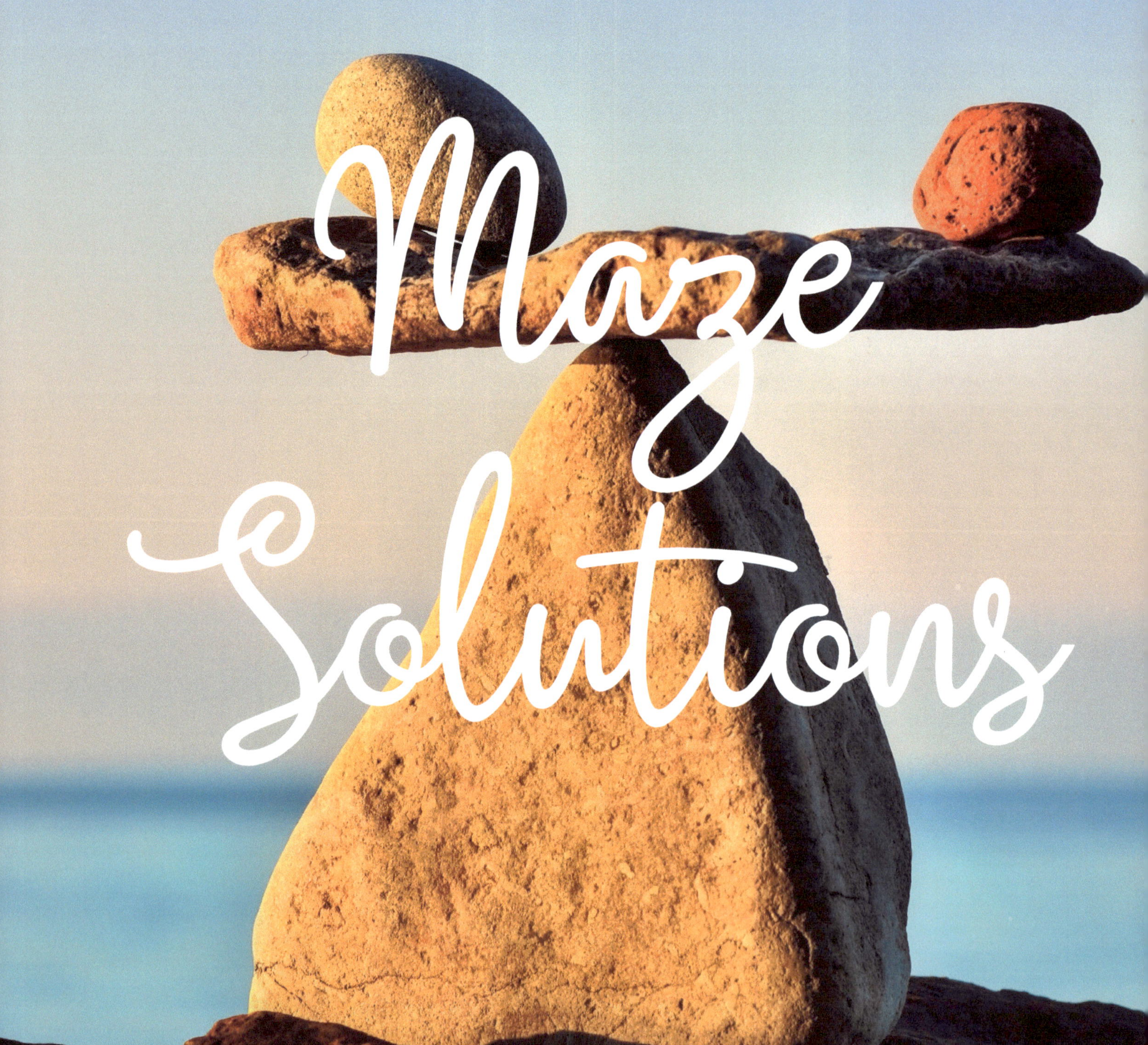

Maze
Solutions

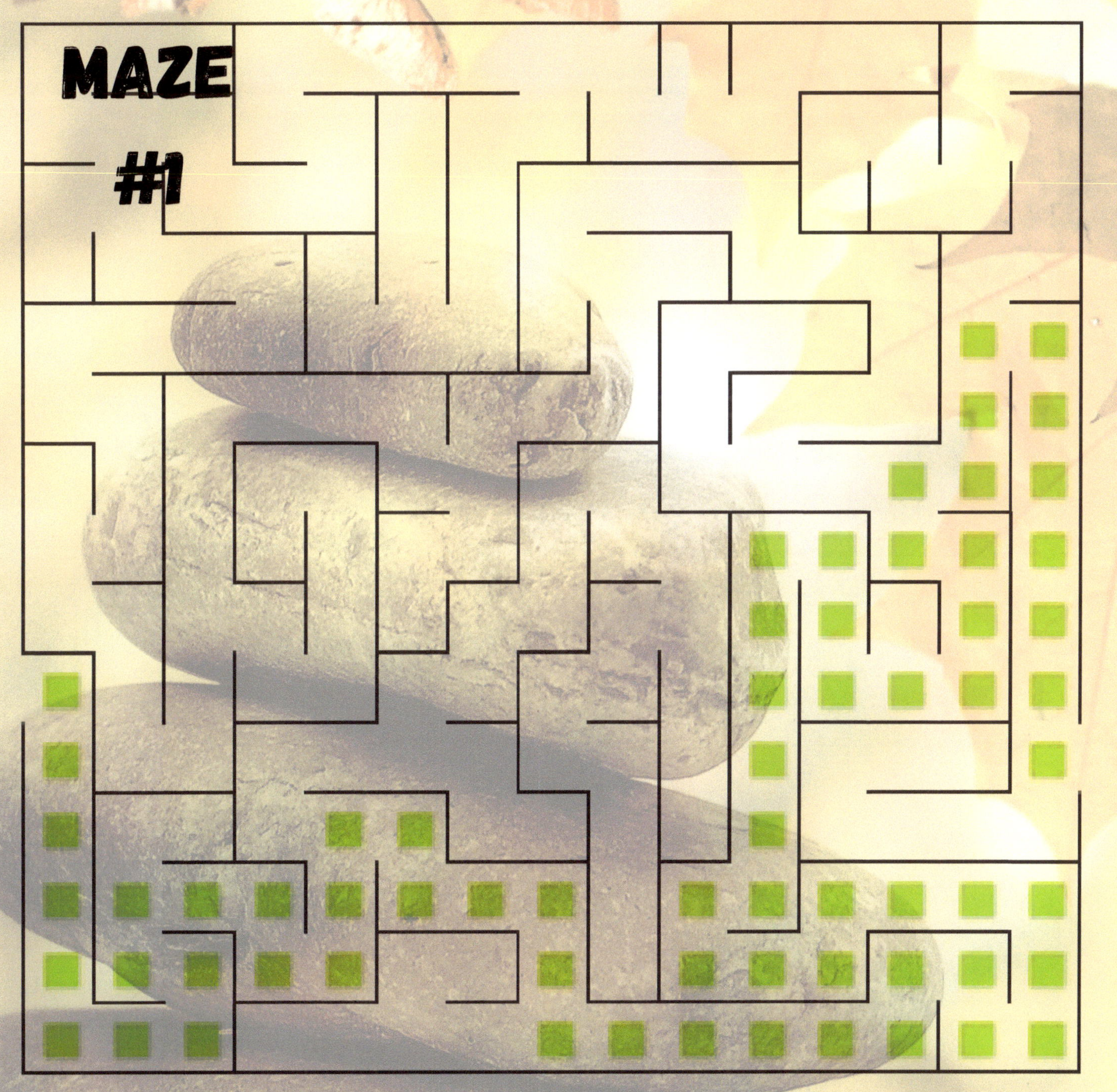
MAZE
#1

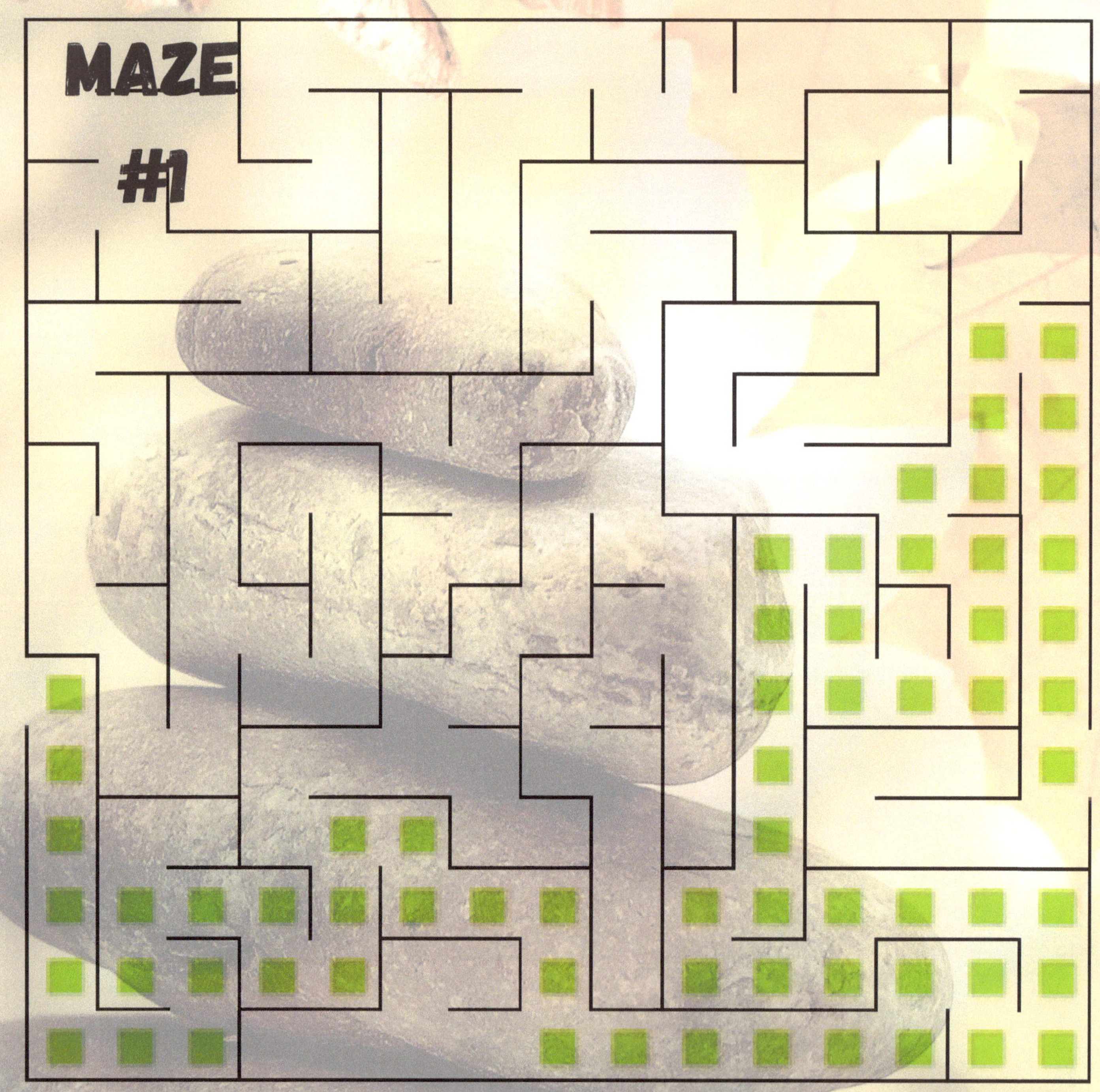

MAZE
#1

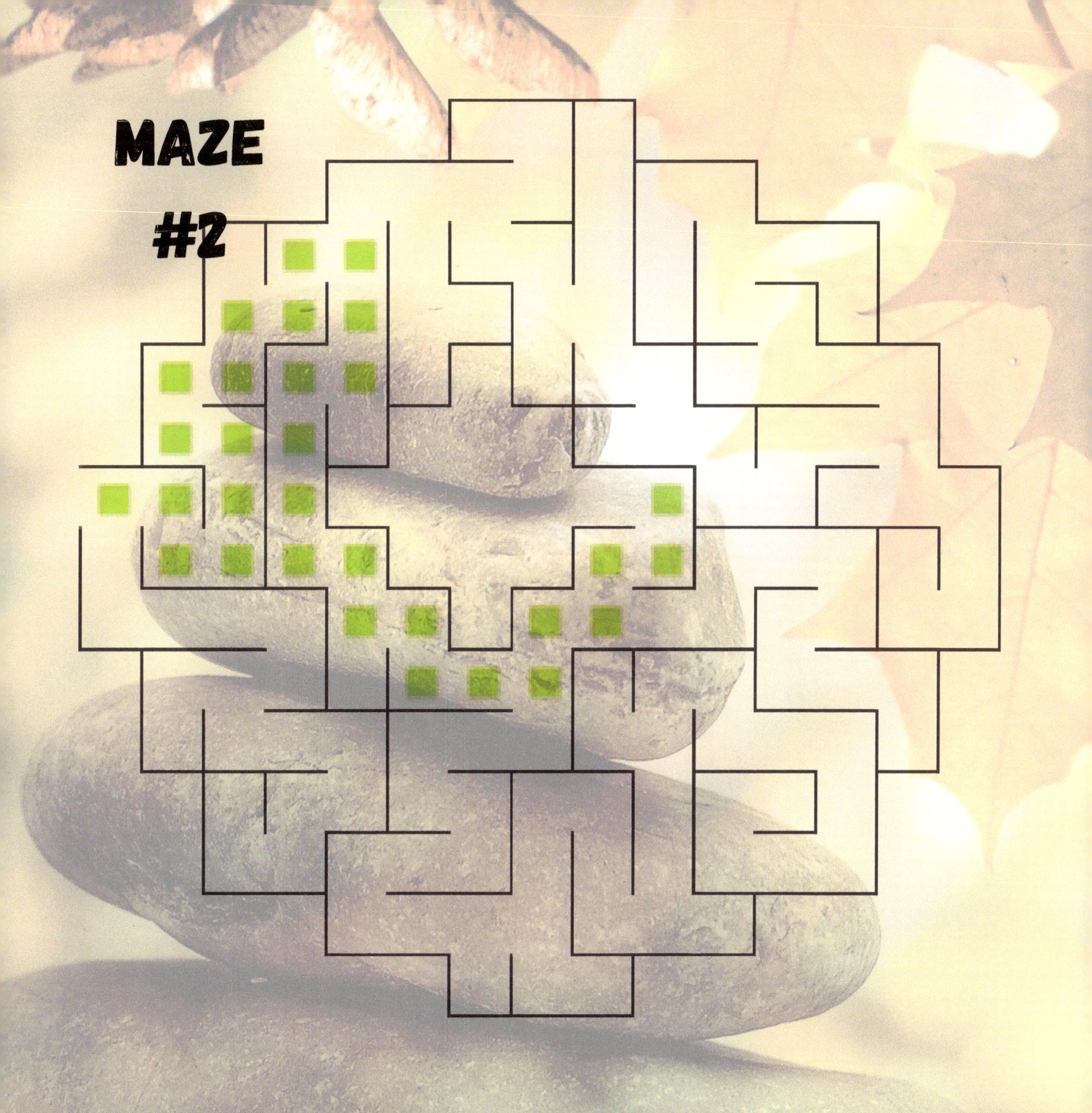

MAZE
#2

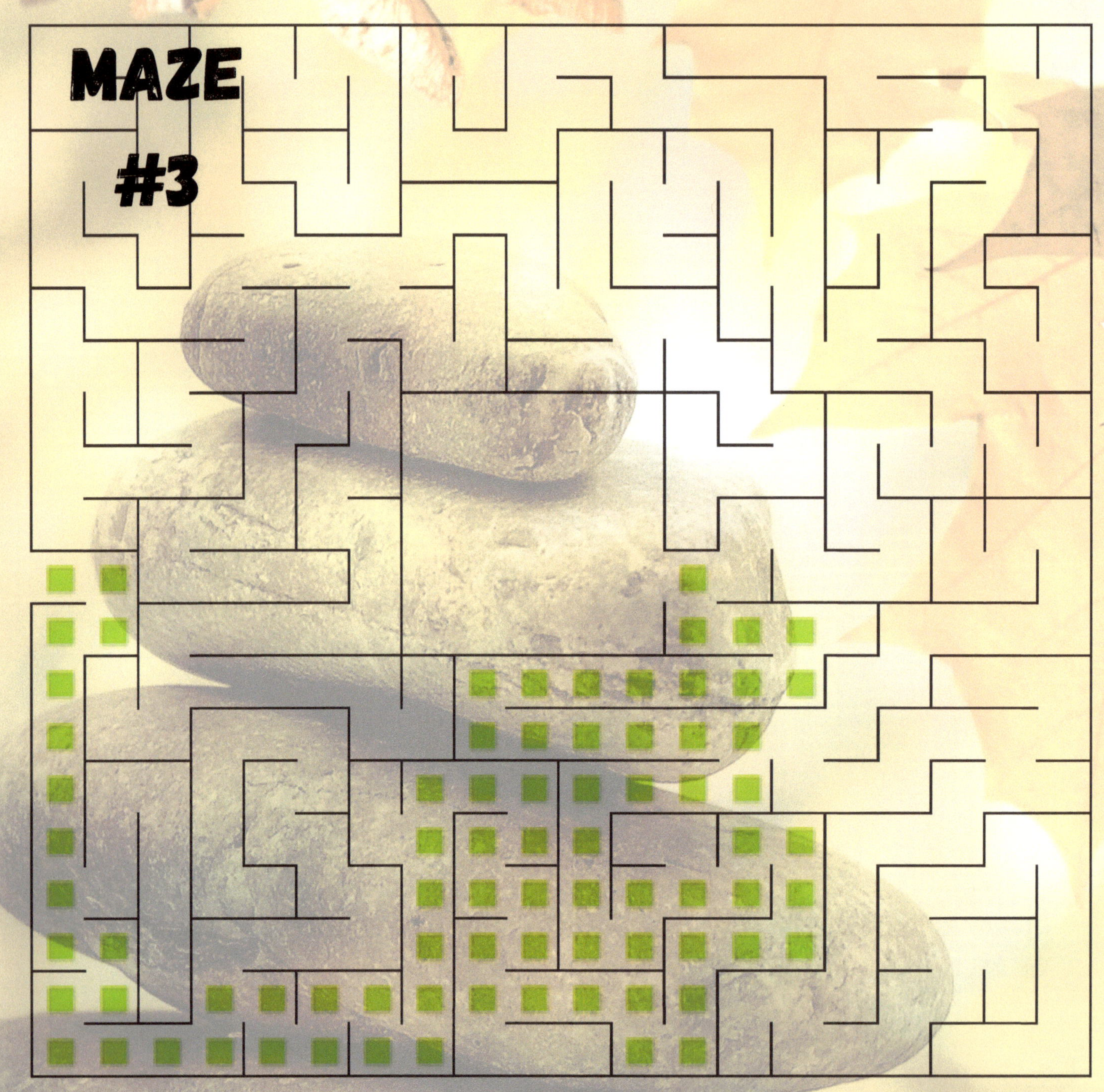

MAZE
#3

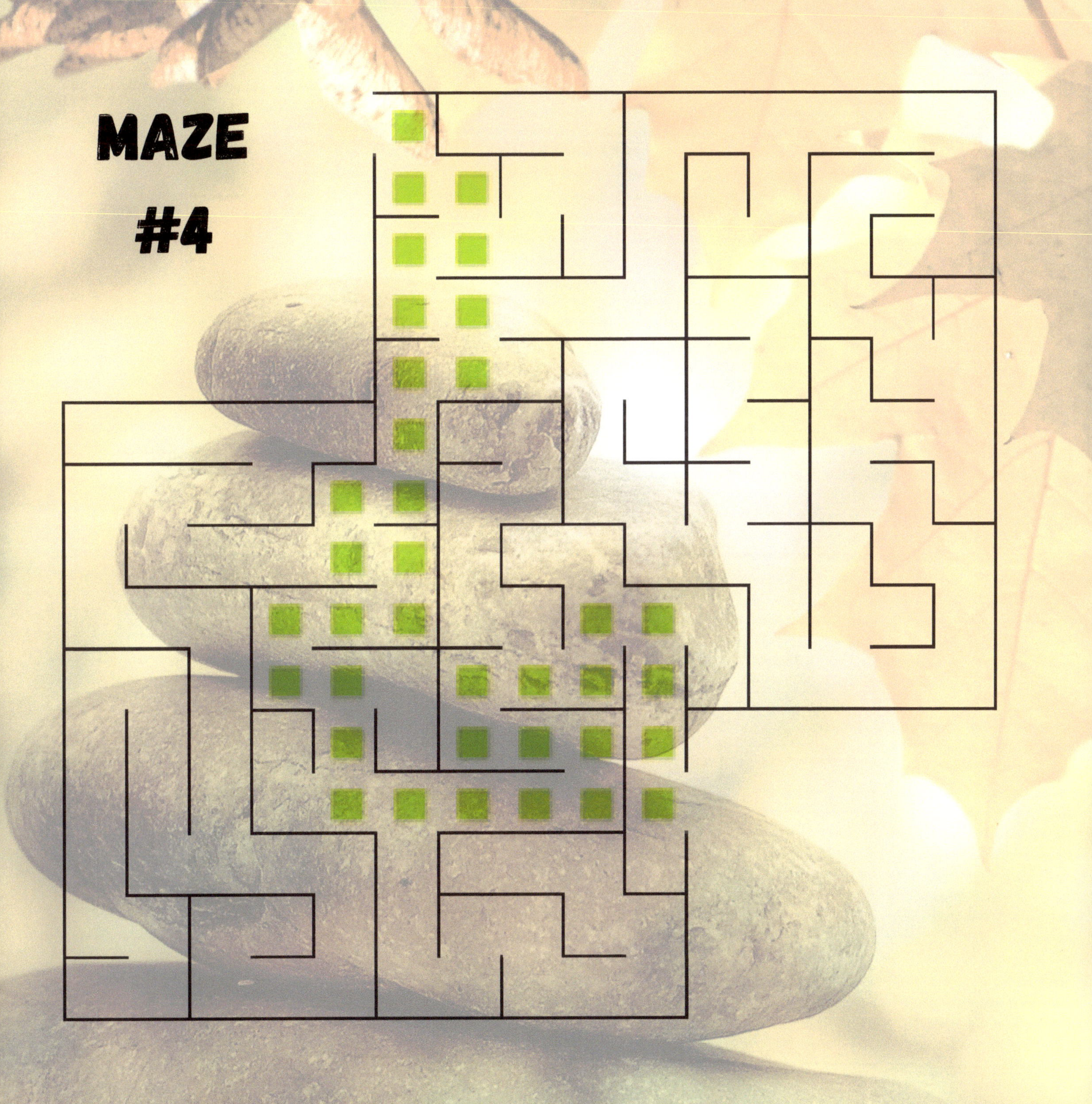

MAZE
#4

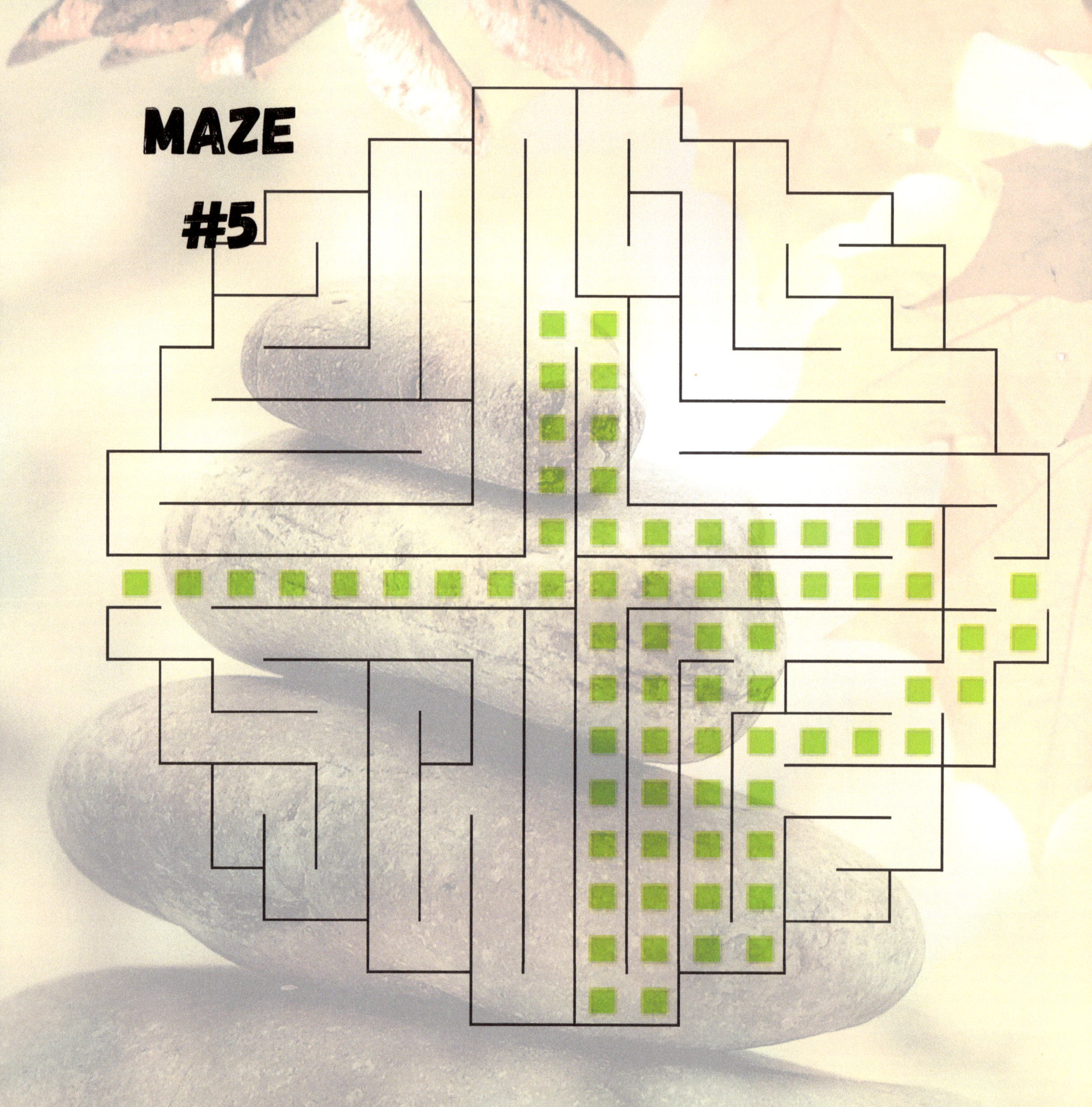

MAZE
#5

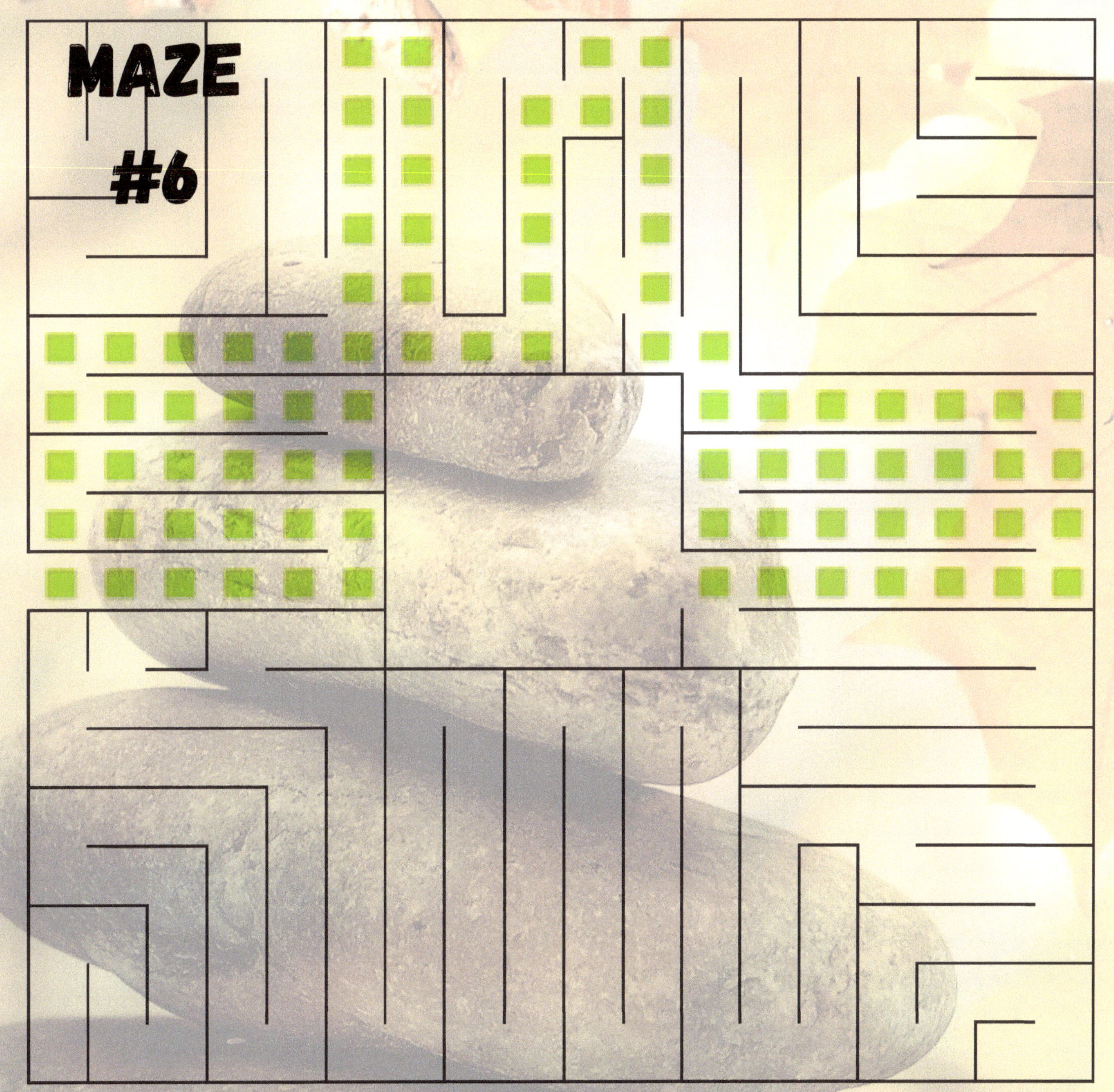

MAZE
#6

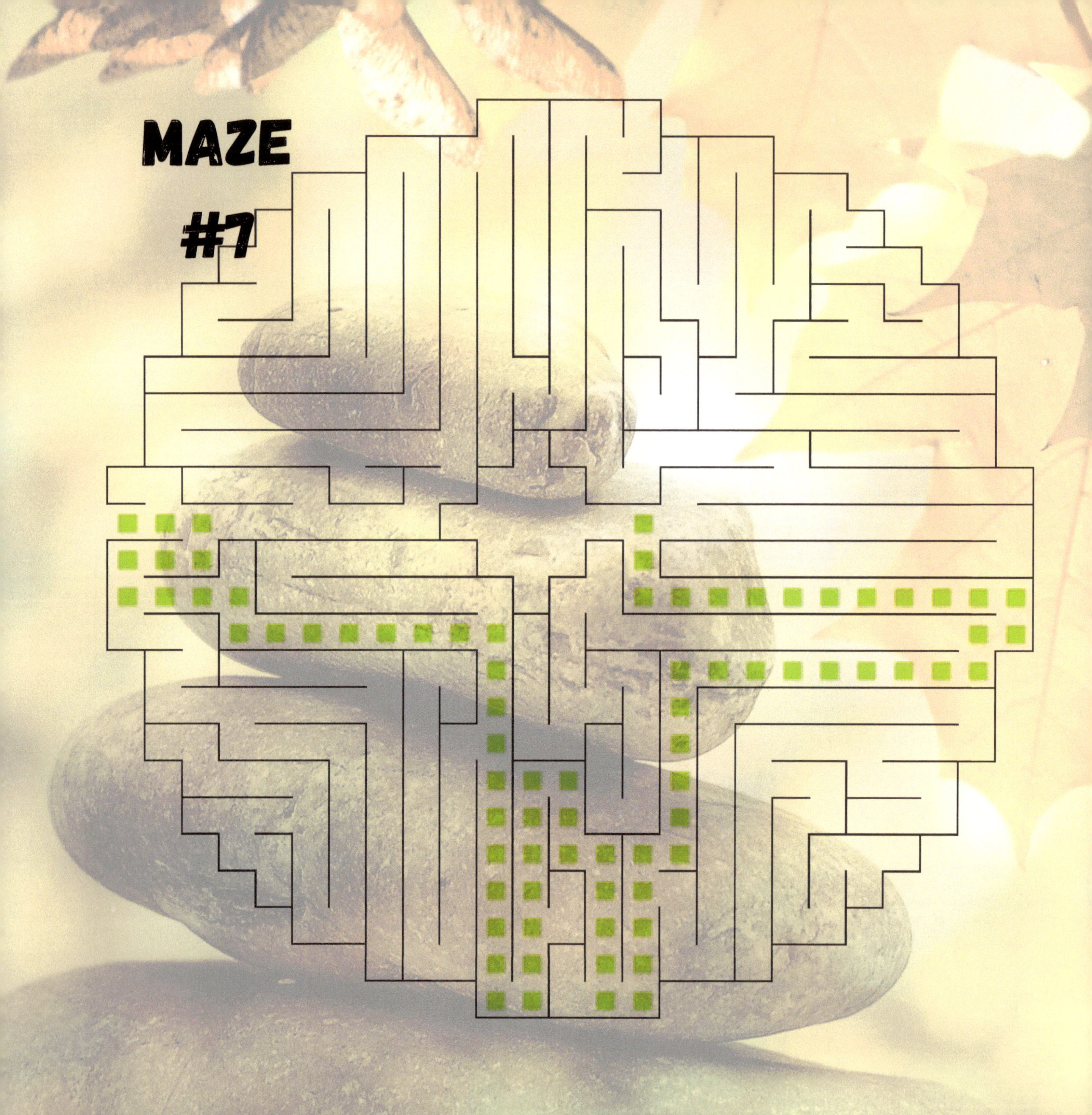
MAZE
#7

MAZE

#8

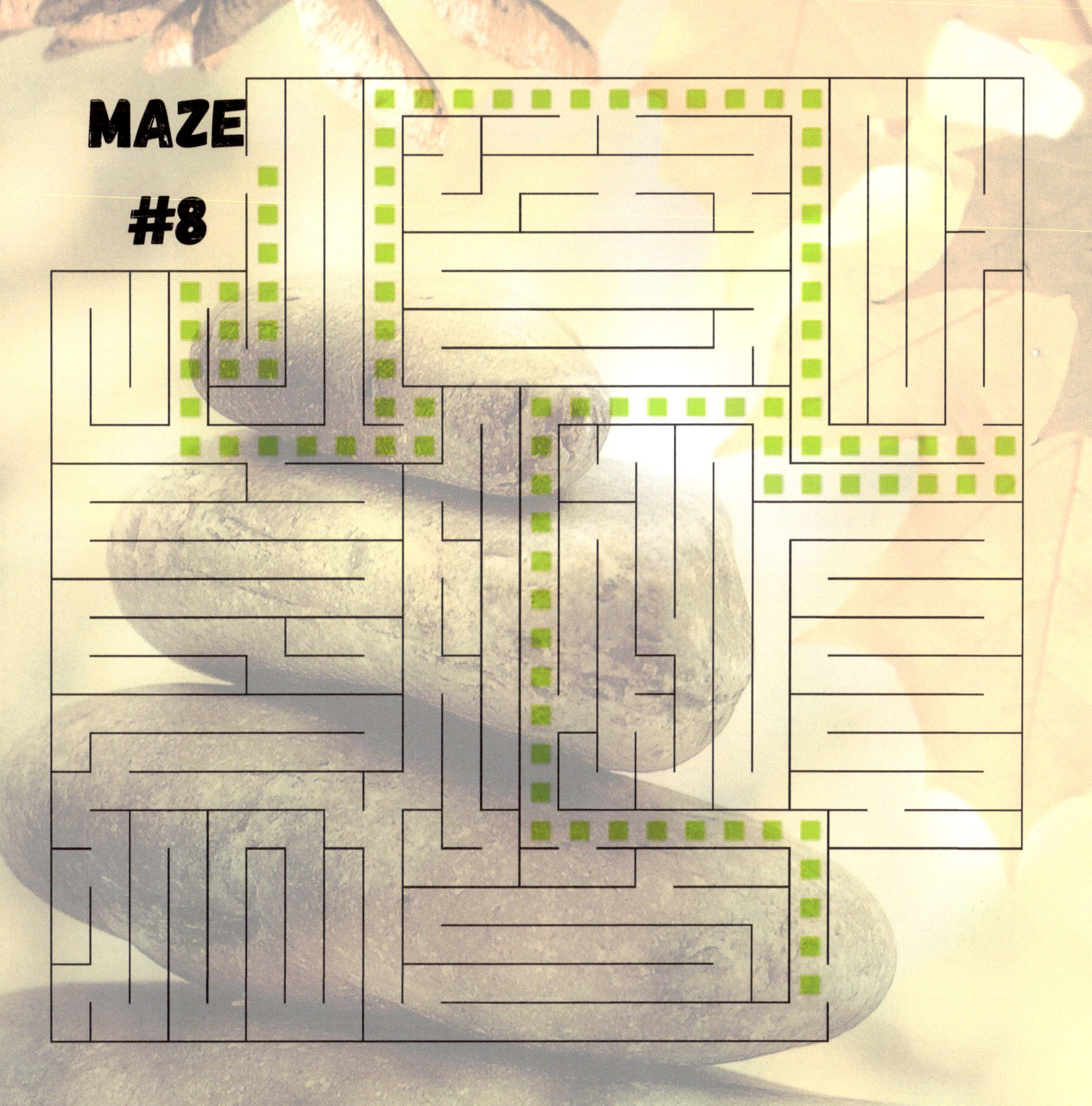

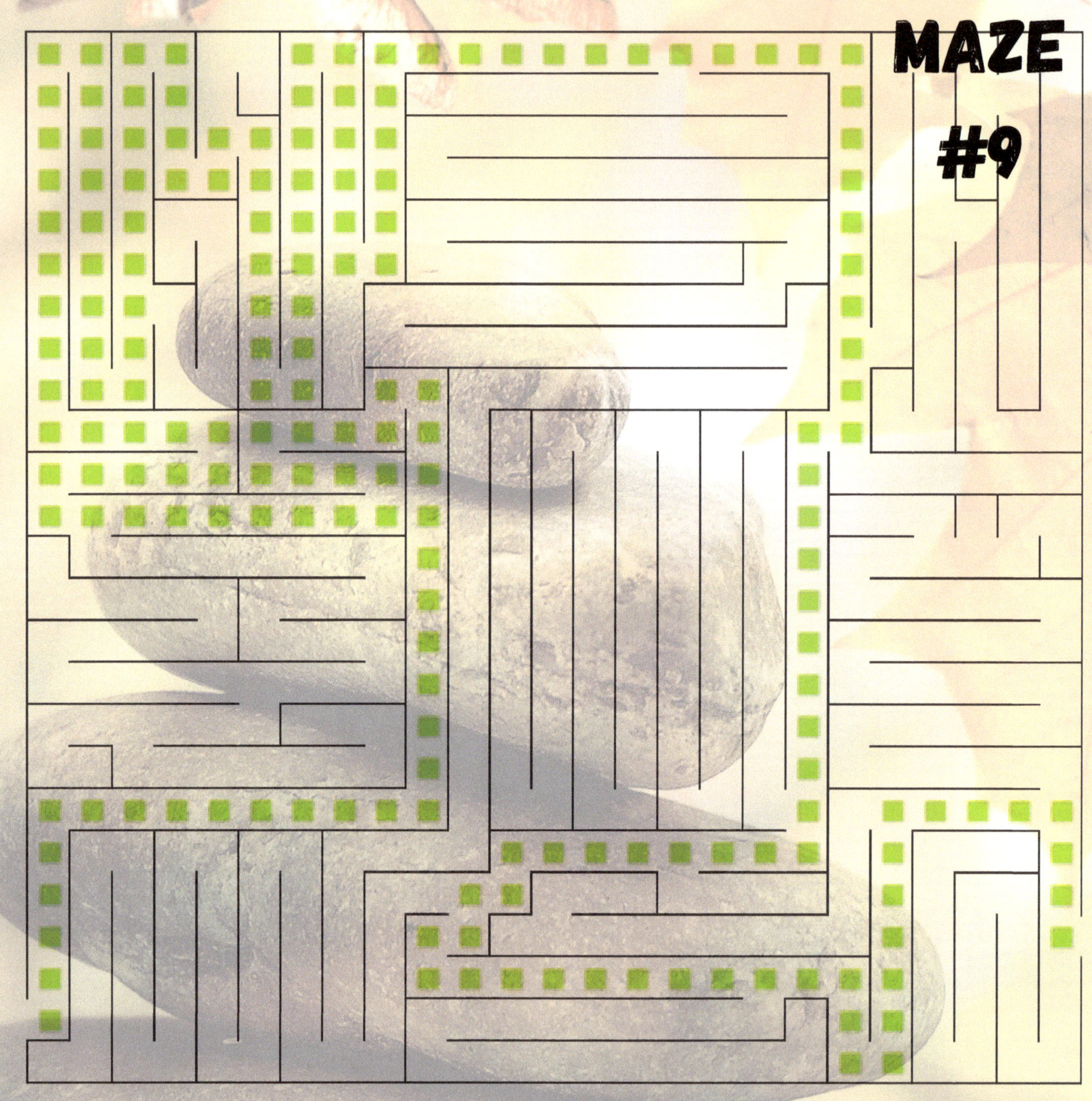

MAZE
#9

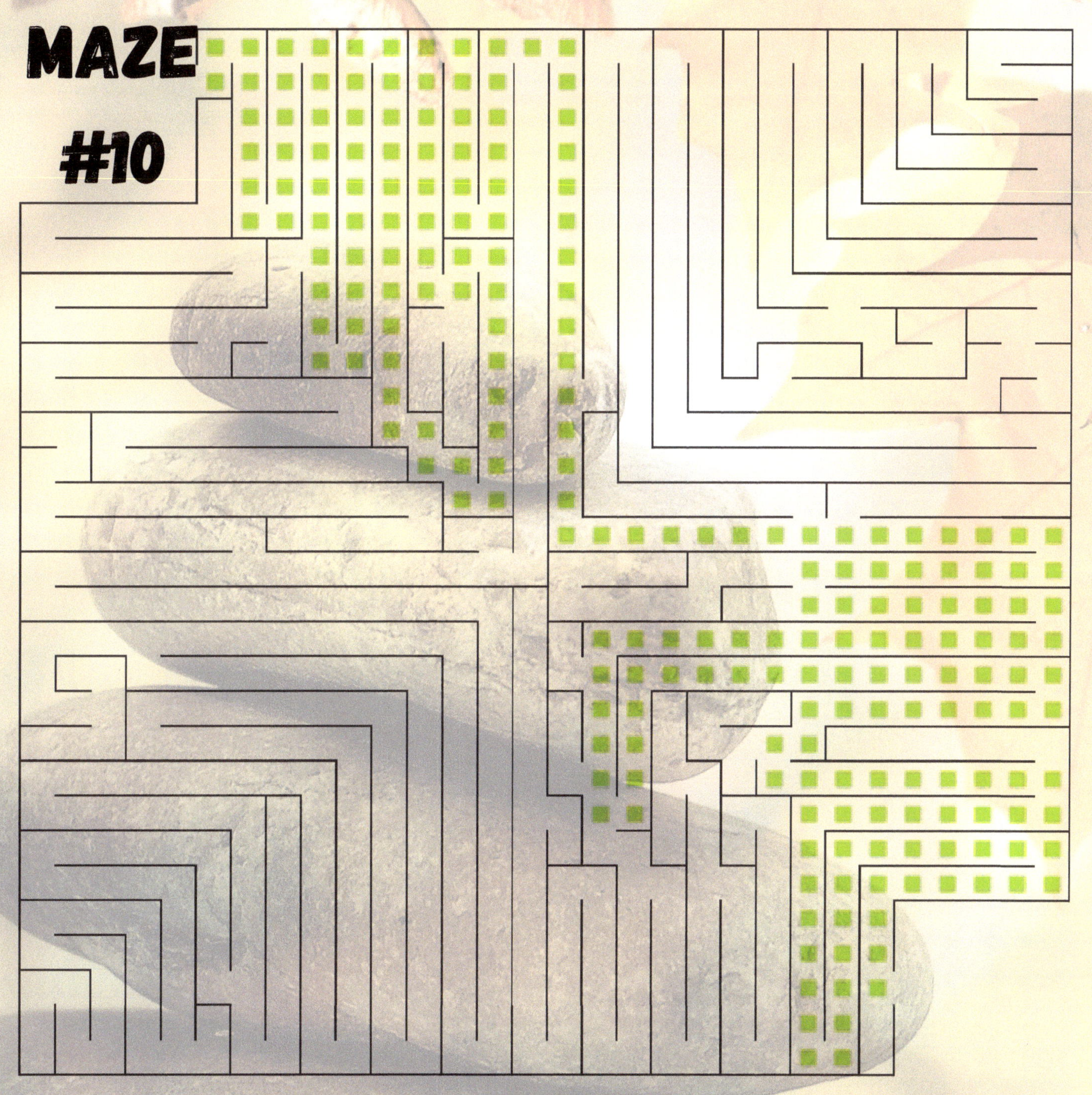

MAZE
#10

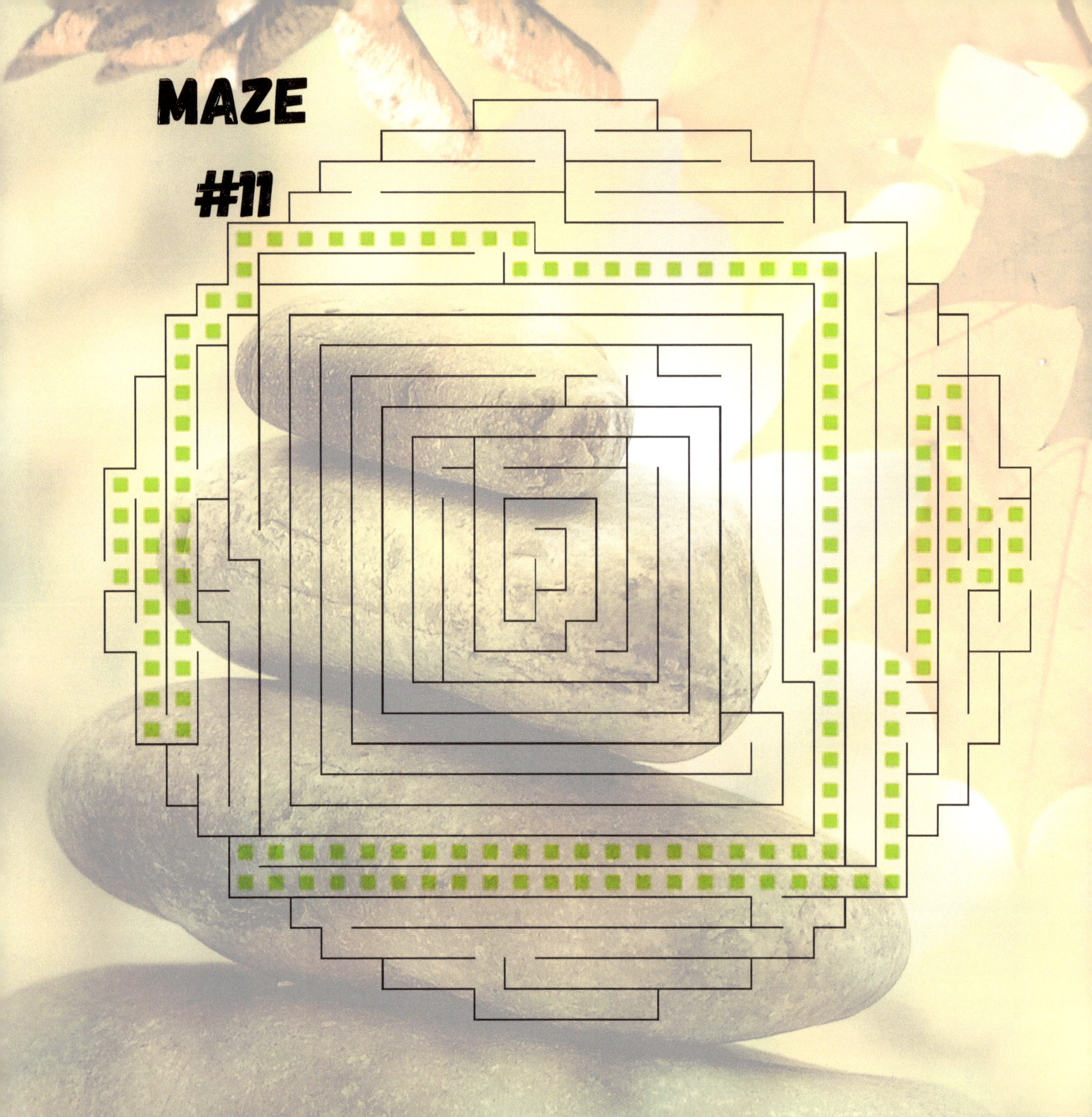
MAZE
#11

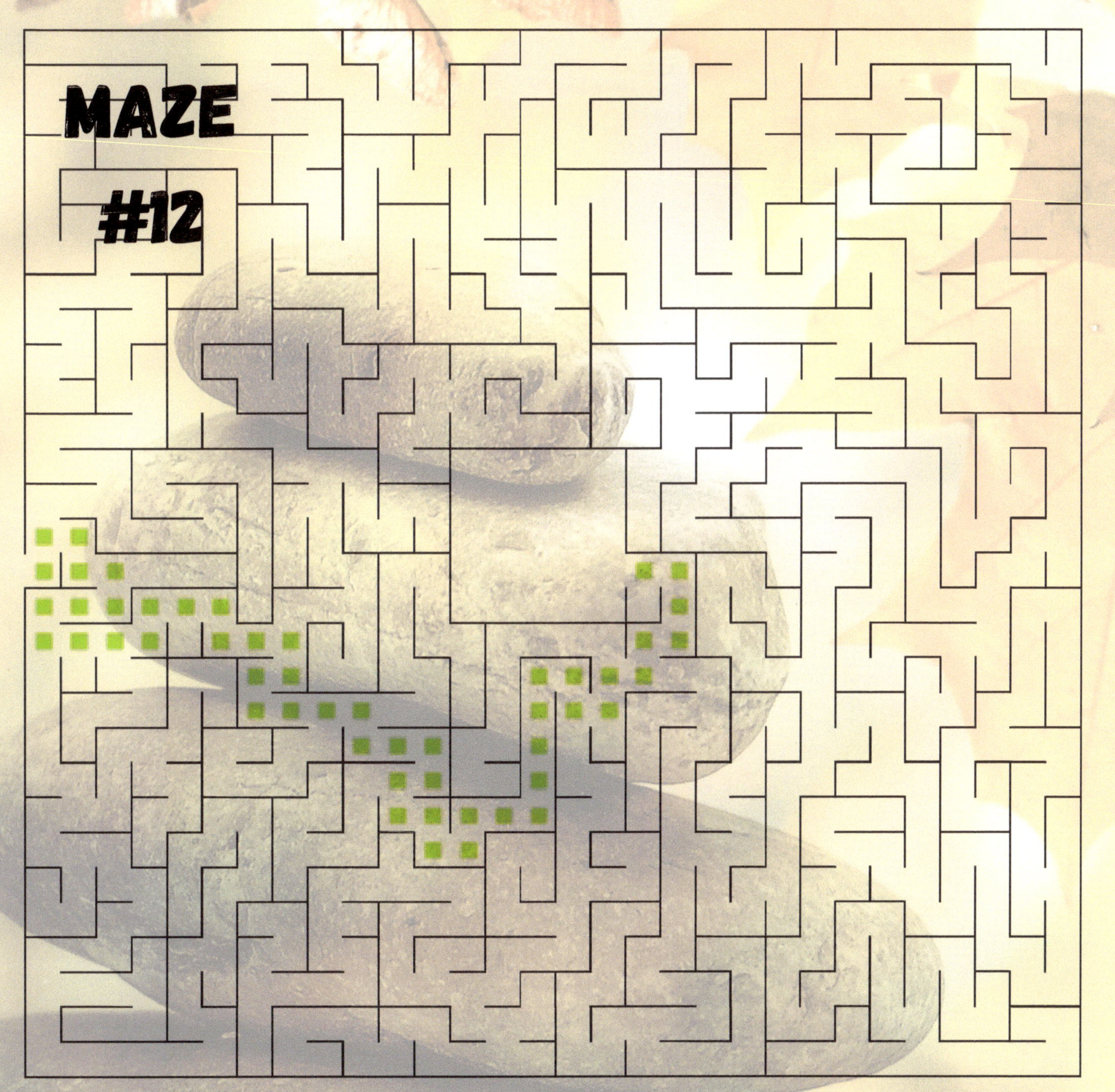

MAZE
#12